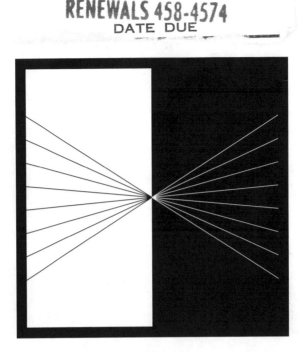

COMMUNITY HEALTH
INFORMATION SYSTEMS
Lessons for the Future

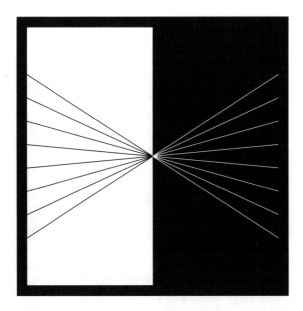

COMMUNITY HEALTH
INFORMATION SYSTEMS
Lessons for the Future

KAREN A. DUNCAN

02 01 00 99 98   5 4 3 2 1

Library of Congress Cataloging-in-Publication Data

Duncan, K. A. (Karen A.)
    Community health information systems : lessons for the future / Karen A. Duncan.
        p.   cm.
    Includes bibliographical references and index.
    ISBN 1-56793-071-9 (alk. paper)
        1. Information storage and retrieval systems—Health services administration.   2. Information storage and retrieval systems—Community health services.   3. Information storage and retrieval systems—Medical care.   I. Title.
    RA971.6.D83   1997   97-39549
    25.06'36212—dc21   CIP

The paper used in this publication meets the minimum requirements of American National Standard for Information Sciences—Permanence of Paper for Printed Library Materials, ANSI Z39.48-1984. ∞ ™

Health Administration Press
A division of the Foundation
    of the American College of
    Healthcare Executives
One North Franklin
Suite 1700
Chicago, IL 60606
312/424-2800

For my loving and beloved mother,
who reads everything I write.

Contents

List of Illustrations

Table of Acronyms

AHCPR   Agency for Health Care Policy and Research
CDR   Central data repository
CHIN   Community health information network
CHIP   CHIN in progress
CHIS   Community health information system
CHMIS   [John A. Hartford Foundation's] Community Health Management Information System
CISC   Community information service centers
CMPI   Community master patient index
COMNET   Community Medical Network [Society]
CPR   Computer-based patient record
CPRI   Computer-based Patient Record Institute
DRG   Diagnosis related group
HCFA   Health Care Financing Administration
HEDIS   Health Plan Employer Data and Information Set
HIN   Health information network
HMO   Health maintenance organization
HPCC   High performance computing and communications program
IT   Information technology
JCAHO   Joint Commission on Accreditation of Healthcare Organizations
MCO   Managed care organization
MKB   Medical knowledge base
MPI   Master patient index
MSA   Medical savings account
NCQA   National Committee for Quality Assurance

NHIS	National health information system
NII	National information infrastructure
PPO	Preferred provider organization
PSRO	Professional Standards Review Organization
RHIS	Regional health information system
VSP	Value-added service provider
WAN	Wide area network
WHIN	Wisconsin Health Information Network

Foreword

I agreed to write this foreword after I had planned a business trip to Paris; it was there that I organized my thoughts for it. It should come as no surprise that I found myself in a philosophic frame of mind as I landed in France. I began thinking of different ideals that the French and American cultures have traditionally held high. And it was in this context that I briefly considered the challenges facing the healthcare industry and business in general.

Take France as an example. Like several other countries, France is attempting to do business within the framework of the European Community. Thus far, the experience has been marked by distrust and suspicion. France remains mindful of other members' motives and hesitates in engaging fully (a feeling and attitude shared by other countries). There is a fear of losing individuality by committing to a whole. I had to wonder where the spirit of *Liberté, Equalité, and Fraternité* fits in here.

And I thought about the United States. An article on the front page of the newspaper reports that U.S. healthcare is failing most of the time in its effort to insure more of its people. Statistics point to increasing costs, decreasing coverage, and a widening in the gap between the insured and the uninsured. Merger mania has eased for now as the largest for-profit healthcare system restructures in the face of a government investigation into possible reimbursement fraud. *Freedom and Justice for All?* I could figure this one out.

I did not end up thinking all is lost. Luckily for us, there are always those individuals who keep the faith.

Ten years ago, technology innovators, medical professionals, and consumer advocates realized that certain technological advances could have a positive effect on the healthcare industry. The potential would exist for unaffiliated stakeholders of the healthcare delivery system to collaborate and share information in a standardized electronic format. From 1992 to 1996, the Community Medical Network (ComNet) Society tracked the growth and fostered the development of health information networks, the necessary framework for the Community Health Information Network (CHIN). As a founder and CEO of this not-for-profit organization, I was privileged to be a spokesperson for the CHIN movement and to have a front row seat for watching its progress.

The movement was at its peak when Karen Duncan began communicating with ComNet to gather information for this book. I am gratified by her work. She has chronicled the movement's rise and fall, has identified lessons learned, and has made valuable comments on future possibilities.

For myself, having lived through the healthcare technology revolution, I have left behind my diary and notes for others to consider and have moved to another arena. Although Karen has certainly been thorough in stating the issues, benefits, barriers, and results of the CHIN movement, she has also provided me an opportunity to share a few personal observations:

- Energy is a living thing, not static but kinetic. Our technology development is mirroring human systems of learning and communicating.

- Knowledge is power, personal power. Control of healthcare information is an attempt by one stakeholder group to block another, so it can gain the personal power to inhibit life's natural flow.

- Internet technology and web access are enabling us to adapt to the evolutionary patterns for acquiring knowledge. It has ended the debate over communication and data standards.

- The concept of gaining access to and sharing healthcare information took a big step backward during the stage of catch-up required by healthcare organizations to build the new technological "infostructures," create the business incentives, and deal with the ramifications of merger and acquisition. With these in place, can we now get past the competitive barriers?

I believe that we can build a stronger nation and come closer to our ideals by empowering individuals to access information, seek knowledge, and assume responsibility for the care of their own health. Further, we must align private and public agendas if we are ever to achieve a healthier planet. Karen challenges the industry to end the "information isolation."

I want to recognize the American College of Healthcare Executives for supporting the publication of this book and for asking me to write the foreword. This professional association has shown its commitment to bringing relevant issues—even if they are not the most popular ones—to the attention of busy healthcare executives.

And finally, thank you, Karen, for a job well done. Only time will tell if the technology that led to the CHIN movement will be used for the good of healthcare around the world.

Pamela I. Hanlon, FACHE, M.B.A., S.T.M.
Former Vice-President, Business Development,
Integrated Medical Systems, Inc.
Founder and Former CEO, Community Medical
Network (ComNet) Society
Professor of Sacred Theology and Doctoral Candidate,
American Apostolic University

Preface

This book was written for healthcare executives who want to be sure that information technology investments made today will grow in value tomorrow, and that their information systems will insulate their enterprises from the expense and burden of changing organizational boundaries and shifting physician and patient populations. It is written also for executives who understand that the best healthcare enterprises are those that directly serve healthcare needs and goals. Fortunately, the same information systems that serve an enterprise's need to survive and thrive can also serve the healthcare needs of the community.

All healthcare enterprises, whether provider or plan, need much more accomplished information systems than they have now. In addition to their potential for administrative simplification, the primary goals driving future health information systems will be

- to measure and report the quality of care to consumers, purchasers, payors, regulators, and accreditors; and
- to achieve the highest level of care possible, given current medical knowledge.

Both of these drivers will require sophisticated, widely accessible information systems that integrate computer-based patient records spanning the continuum of care, with data repositories and tools for the clinical guidance of healthcare professionals.

Moving ahead in either the quality or the administrative arena requires systems that can reach beyond institutional walls; neither can be implemented effectively with in-house systems alone. Healthcare executives have recognized that they must collaborate in creating communitywide information systems if they expect to achieve the information flows they need to compete. As a result, hundreds of healthcare enterprises throughout the United States have participated in developing community health information networks (CHINs) that make essential healthcare information accessible.

But CHINs have not yet lived up to their promise. Indeed, it may be possible for them to do so only after the ideas and purposes that underpin CHINs are reexamined. CHINs have fallen behind in development; they have exceeded their budgets; and they have lost substantial participant support. Recovering the ground lost depends on searching for lessons, and then on understanding and acting on those lessons. This book was born of that reexamination, which in turn has led to the inescapable conclusion that we need to alter perspectives about what CHINs can accomplish, and then change the climate for CHINs so they can work their magic.

The key flaw in today's CHINs is the failure of their initiators to plan strategically. Instead of asking, "What can I do with information technology to solve important healthcare problems?", the question has been "What do I need to promise in order to justify a CHIN?" While most CHINs have laudable goals such as improving the quality of healthcare, many fail to actually plan for and develop capabilities that have genuine relevance to these goals. In fact, many CHINs initially implement—at great expense—rudimentary communications capabilities that do not solve healthcare system problems and in fact verge on complicating providers' lives rather than improving them. Many CHINs appear to be accomplishing little more than automating or replacing existing processes that already work, rather than opening up vital and valuable new information flows.

The most serious results of this inattention to relevance are

- failure to obtain sufficient support and participation by over-selling CHIN capabilities, while at the same time underselling the potential value of CHIN applications; and

- crises of confidence stemming from nonalignment of mission among participants and other stakeholders who are or should be benefiting from the CHIN.

This book explains how CHINs sink into the unhappy consequences of overselling the value and relevance of their capabilities, and failing to perceive and communicate the rich CHIN potential. To stimulate fresh thinking about what CHINs actually should be doing for a community, numerous scenarios of relatively uncomplex CHINs designed to solve serious community healthcare problems appear throughout. This kind of focus is recommended for creating successful, durable CHINs. Such CHINs not only will support healthcare interests, but will also attract support from throughout the community, including non-healthcare businesses and organizations. They will attract support in ways that administrative simplification simply cannot because it does not serve the community.

The book also describes approaches to strategic planning for CHIN initiators that will avoid later crises of confidence. Those in charge can strategize successfully by making a commitment to goal-focused development and by applying simple techniques that ensure the relevance of planned CHIN capabilities to the healthcare goals of CHIN participants. Essential principles and useful techniques are both explained.

Three of these principles seem deceptively simple, but they clearly need reinforcement:

- the principle of the practical value of goal consensus;
- the principle of cooperating in order to compete more effectively; and
- the principle of leveraging CHIN assets across applications.

Following models in the book, healthcare executives must use these principles to justify CHINs by focusing directly on healthcare system problems that transcend institutional boundaries. In this way, they ensure that their systems will continue to serve effectively through these turbulent times and beyond.

In the not-too-distant future, when CHINs are fully developed and integrated into every aspect of healthcare, the networks will no longer be called CHINs, but CHIS—community health information *systems* fully able to serve as a true information infrastructure and partner for the healthcare system.

Barriers to development of a true CHIS can be found in many quarters in addition to the CHIN itself and its participants. Few technology barriers still exist, but daunting cultural barriers remain to prevent the rich CHIN potential from being realized. Healthcare executives are in the best position to break down these cultural barriers. They can work as CHIN advocates through professional associations, legislation, and regulation to end the culture of information isolation in healthcare, where every provider keeps private records incompatible in format and content with virtually all other providers. Fresh clinical data of high quality are badly needed, not only for clinical quality assessment, but also to fuel clinical research that can help close the yawning gaps in medical knowledge and clinical practice.

In their own organizations, healthcare executives have the power to end the rapid proliferation of private information systems that perpetuate information isolation and, instead, to commit resources to cooperative systems. They can lead their organizations in a commitment to cooperative development and adoption of essential standards and protocols for information specification and sharing, secure telecommunications, and protection of patient and institutional privacy.

Healthcare executives are in a unique position to change the community perspective about CHINs and ultimately CHISs. But they must think in terms of collaborative solutions and value-added services, reaching into all corners, including schools, businesses, community groups, and government agencies. They can imaginatively and proactively assess their community's potential for good health and quality healthcare, and then generate the excitement that gaining a CHIN well deserves. In the community, they can ask: Who does not have access to care? What are the health threats? What medical problems are not as well managed as they should be? Is there a better way to organize care? Given our finite resources, how can community healthcare enterprises work together to maximize service?

Healthcare executives who recognize these questions as the most important ones they can ask will find in this book an ally in bringing to life CHINs and CHISs that cross institutional boundaries to respond to community needs, and that also serve increasingly complex enterprise needs for external information flow. By their fundamental nature such systems would protect enterprises from the pendulum swings of styles of healthcare organization and payment. CHINs and CHISs that accommodate, support, and transcend such changes will continue to serve their participant enterprises and communities well into the nascent postmodern healthcare era.

LOOKING BACK AT CHINS

I n the early 1990s, a happy convergence occurred: appropriate information technology caught up with the need for a greatly enhanced flow of information throughout the healthcare system. The tools of information technology had become available and affordable, and healthcare executives were ready to embrace them. This achievement triggered a nationwide burst of interinstitutional information network development: the Community Health Information Network (CHIN) phenomenon. Collectively known as CHINs, these networks represented a first step to collaboration among healthcare enterprises in creating a shared information infrastructure that would improve service and reduce the cost of doing business.

By 1995, some 500 CHINs were in operation, development, or planning stages (Community Medical Network Society 1995). According to the Community Medical Network (COMNET) Society, the CHINs were to be used initially and primarily for administrative purposes. Other early priorities, in order of popularity, were clinical, financial, and educational applications and the use of CHINs as data repositories. But it soon became clear that CHINs had a lot to offer beyond the readily apparent or easily described early uses. In the short span of their existence to date, they had become many different things to many people. They were to become a symbol of the hopes and dreams of healthcare professionals everywhere.

Healthcare providers and payors especially, in common with officials in many of the nation's complex industries such as banking and the airlines, recognized that collaborative use of information technology held the key to more efficient operation and better service —and to profitability.

Clinical informaticians were ecstatic. Their 40 years of missionary work, spent spreading the word about the consummate need for the computer-based patient record, were finally beginning to pay off. Information technology had freed the administrative and financial functions of healthcare institutions from the tyranny of information flow limitations within the institution. Now, if information could begin to flow among healthcare institutions—if those institutions could share medical records—clinical medicine could also be transformed. A single electronic medical record would be recognized at last as the essential building block of the future networked healthcare system, and its potential for patient benefit would be realized.

Futurists, too, saw their visions about to be confirmed. CHINs would be the first step toward using technology to finally and fully integrate the disparate parts of the healthcare system, both internally and externally with the overall healthcare environment. CHINs could make transformation possible along the vertical continuum of care among disparate enterprises as well as the horizontal continuum of clinical care, professional and consumer education, research, management, and policy. Even better, CHINs could lead to a more practical yet more fulfilling redefinition of the paths to good health and could even transform our very concepts of time and space in healthcare—where it would be provided, how it would be delivered, and who would deliver it. Such achievements would require cooperation and collaboration on a national scale, including and affecting every provider and every patient in the healthcare system. Futurists viewed the CHIN movement as a welcome shift in attitude—perhaps even as a maturation of understanding—with local efforts in the form of CHINs serving as the essential first step.

Since 1995, however, CHIN initiatives have slowed, and many projects established have been scaled back or postponed. Paradoxically, this step backward for the CHIN phenomenon comes at a time when virtually all other industries in the United States are seeking ways to expand their uses of information technology (IT). Clearly, the cyberworld of ubiquitous computing and networking is fast approaching for all industries. In healthcare, the value of information technology to the successful future of the system is not in doubt. The need for a better flow of information is overwhelming, and the task is too great to be tackled by individual enterprises. Community partnerships are essential to the creation of electronic information flows. The value of community collaboration is undiminished by the fact that some CHIN efforts have stumbled on the first step. Despite the early difficulties, it seems clear that

CHINs or other CHIN-like networks are the information conduits of the future.

This book focuses on the benefits envisioned in bringing CHINs to a community and on the strategies needed to achieve those objectives. If CHIN planners and initiators have not been achieving their goals, it is because their strategic planning has fallen short. They have failed to take into account and to incorporate into their planning the role of health information networks, especially CHINs, in the future of healthcare. They have failed to set realistic goals that are in tune with the needs of the healthcare system and the community itself. And they have failed to plan in ways consistent with those goals and even, in many cases, with their own CHIN objectives. The subsequent dissonance within CHINs has been daunting and can be overcome only by taking the missing goal-reconciling steps.

The task of this book is to direct the attention of healthcare executives to these problems of CHIN strategy: What are they? How and why do they occur? How can we remedy them? Such problems can be untangled now and avoided in the future using several simple tools described in these pages.

Given the juxtaposition of the importance of collaborative networking and its apparent difficulties, it seems reasonable to consider contemporary CHINs as perhaps the early stages in the continuum of maturation of collaborative concepts and projects. So the question for healthcare is not whether to develop health information networks, including CHINs, but rather, who will conceptualize the future and control the systems design, development, and information flow for healthcare, and how can healthcare executives ensure orderly and optimal development?

All healthcare professionals, whether or not they are associated with a CHIN, should understand the philosophy and concepts underlying CHINs and should learn from what has happened with CHINs over the past few years. Healthcare executives who are involved with CHINs now have already made a considerable investment and want to maximize its value. Those not involved with CHINs yet should learn from those who are, thus avoiding as many potential problems as possible. Clinical informaticians who need CHINs to advance the art and science of clinical medicine must prepare themselves for a leadership role in CHIN development. No group, whether provider, payor, purchaser, patient, or public interest, will be able for long to remain aloof from health information networking.

As a prelude to learning from the past, this chapter describes a CHIN in all of its variety, briefly reviews milestones in CHIN history, and then points to succeeding chapters in which specific CHIN problems are examined and solutions proposed.

WHAT IS A CHIN?

Understanding the history of CHINs begins with coming to a common idea of what a CHIN is and is not. Early definitions of CHINs, including the author's, were idealistic, requiring the CHIN to act as a system serving the health information needs of all healthcare stakeholders and making information on the network available to all (Duncan 1995). Since few self-styled CHINs could meet that definition, or were even planning to do so, we should first approach a workable definition by distinguishing between the ideal and the reality.

And this is the reality: a CHIN exists when two or more community organizations create a shared computer network to be used for agreed-upon healthcare purposes. Earlier definitions reflected more the hopes of their authors than could probably be attained in the early stages of CHIN development. Those definitions held the hope that CHINs would achieve an ideal joining together of all community-based healthcare entities to serve the good of the community, rather than just the specific needs of the participants in the CHIN. CHINs almost invariably included the greater scope in their mission statements, but few actually worked toward such goals. Those that had such goals but were far short of achieving them were optimistically termed CHIPs—CHINs-in-Progress (Hanlon 1994).

CHINs in development during the past several years have had in common the ability to move healthcare information beyond the walls of the institution and the enterprise for the benefit of all involved parties. However, they have varied widely in many other respects. Typically, the variations have arisen from one or more of the following elements:

- *Stakeholders.* Any individuals or groups who are affected by the CHIN, such as providers, purchasers, payors, patients, accreditors, policymakers, information systems vendors, or the community itself

- *Enterprises.* CHIN participants whose business is healthcare, including payors (e.g., insurance companies and health plans such as HMOs), providers (e.g., hospitals, clinics, doctors and groups, home care agencies, and treatment centers), and ancillary service providers (laboratories and pharmacies)

- *Ownership and management.* Typically providers, payors, or information system vendors, but also community coalitions, governments, or any other grouping of stakeholders

- *Focus.* Arenas chosen for CHIN development, such as administrative, clinical, marketing, or regulation

- *Size.* Areas ranging from a part of a city to an entire state, with many or few suppliers and users of information
- *Scope.* Comparative complexity of design, functionality, or geography
- *Information technology design.* Usually a centralized or distributed system

Variations in these elements most often have resulted from each community's unique characteristics, resources, and capabilities. They are not fundamental factors in the successful implementation of the CHIN, as the chapters that follow explain.

CHINS IN THE BEGINNING

The early impetus for CHINS had little to do with a reasoned, thorough analysis of their potential role in community health and healthcare or of the means to achieve that role. Structural changes in the healthcare environment were driving the demand for information. Payors needed information to analyze outcomes and compare treatment plans. Integrated delivery systems, which combined hospitals, clinics, and other outpatient and subacute care services, needed to share information across their units to reduce overhead and assure continuity of care. The Internet was new and exciting, and so was networking in general, because the technology had finally caught up with people's imaginations.

Insurance companies were among the first significant CHIN players. Their sponsorship of CHINs could leverage their significant enterprise investments in information technology and their sizable claims databases by making these assets more widely available through CHINs for claims processing and analysis. The first real CHIN, the Wisconsin Health Information Network (WHIN), was in fact an enterprise network expanded to include a claims processing relationship with a payor. WHIN offered financial services; communications among various stakeholders, including banks and employers; and clinical information services to hospitals and doctors (Hoban 1995).

The John A. Hartford Foundation's Community Health Management Information System (CHMIS) project was at least partly responsible for the early positive view of CHINs. Begun in 1991, CHMIS' primary goal was to assist communities in addressing the information vacuum, using a transaction system, a database, and a network, to lower healthcare costs and reward quality. The high standards for selection as a CHMIS community, together with the level of planning support available from the Hartford-funded Foundation for Health Care Quality in Seattle, were sufficient to all but guarantee a reasonable measure of success for CHMIS projects.

The Foundation was clear in characterizing the problems the CHMIS project was designed to solve:

> Imagine a shopping center where there are no price tags, where it is impossible to compare merchandise, and where the prices go up 15 to 20% a year without fail. In order to sell their wares, merchants must file a bewildering variety of forms and wait weeks for their money, without knowing how much they will eventually be paid. This, unfortunately, describes our health care system as it is today (John A. Hartford Foundation 1993).

The founding of the COMNET Society in 1993 appeared to mark the successful launching of the CHIN movement. COMNET's laudable goals and programs, designed to bring about "collaborative advancement of enabling, delivery-enhancing infostructures (information infrastructures)," positioned the Society to become an important organizing and unifying force for the 500 CHINs it had identified. But by the end of 1996 the COMNET Society was gone.

WHEN SOMETHING WENT WRONG

In addition to the demise of the COMNET Society, many CHIN organizations were faltering by the mid-90s. Earlier optimism among CHINs was giving way to regrouping and to seeking new direction, new leadership, or both. Several had folded, and the formation of new CHINs had slowed considerably. Something, indeed, had gone wrong.

The turnaround from enthusiasm to apparent disaffection leads to some questions and a search for clues. After all, more than ever— and at a minimum—purchasers need information from payors, payors need information from enterprises, and the public needs information from providers. Are these needs unclear? Has the technology failed to live up to expectations? Have the resources for CHINs been unobtainable? Or has a glimpse of the information-rich future proven to be just too overwhelming for further pursuit?

Three different views offer an important clue to understanding what happened to CHINs. These views, held by distinct segments of the healthcare professional community—healthcare executives, medical informaticians, and futurists—actually represent different *time horizons*—different *horizons of maturity*—for concepts relating to interenterprise information technology networks. Discussions later in this book make it clear that failure to reconcile these views has been a key factor in less-than-successful CHIN implementations.

The *current practical view*, held as the principal view of providers, focuses on information technology used to facilitate existing inter-enterprise or organizational tasks such as authorizations, claims processing, routing of laboratory test results, or telemedicine (in which the healthcare professional and the patient interact from different locations, connected by video or other devices that use telecommunications technology).

The *near-term idealistic view*, espoused primarily by academic and governmental medical informaticians, maintains that the next major breakthrough in medical care will be widespread use of a complete computer-based patient record (CPR). Such a record will be selectively and appropriately available wherever needed and will incorporate all of the information needed for the physician or other health professional to make diagnostic and therapeutic decisions in the best interests of the patient. This information will include both patient-specific data and medical knowledge in the form of guidelines or specific research results. All of a patient's providers, including local or remote hospitals, emergency facilities, clinics, home care providers, pharmacies, testing and treatment centers, schools, and even the patient, will be linked to the CPR to contribute information and make use of it. Only when such a CPR is available can providers achieve a fully formed, longitudinal patient record for use across the continuum of care.

The *transformed future view*, posited by healthcare futurists, accords information the status of a change agent. Currently, virtually all of the information in the healthcare system is trapped, lying useless in file folders or even on computer-generated tape or disk files in unknown, incompatible, or otherwise unusable formats and locations. When this information is flowing appropriately on the information highway, available to entities that previously had no access or that were in locations with no access, the healthcare system will be free to explore expanded concepts of health and new modes of healthcare delivery. For example, if information technology makes medical knowledge available at virtually any location, then paramedical personnel with appropriate skills can provide triage and primary care for patients at, for instance, a network of storefront clinics.

Each of these strikingly different views has in its turn served as the goal for CHINs; together these positions illuminate the difficulty of coming to terms with an accurate definition and an appropriate function for CHINs. Since there is widespread agreement that the technology for CHINs or HINs is ready, and since the need for enhanced information flow is certainly clear, we must look beyond the physical or the tangible to find the path to successful CHINs. A shift in perception is needed. CHIN leaders and healthcare executives need to understand the causes of CHIN problems and then use that information to audit their own CHIN organizations. Heeding these lessons from the past is essential to moving ahead to the next generation of health information systems development, both for existing CHINs and for CHINs whose business plans are not yet finalized.

CARRYING OUT THE PURPOSE OF THIS BOOK

The next two chapters of this book deal with background concepts that lay the groundwork for changing the strategic planning process. Chapter 2 first describes our society's *commonly accepted goals* for healthcare in a way that is convenient for planning. It introduces *systems perspective* as a tool for understanding the immutable relationships that exist in healthcare. A systems perspective is used often in subsequent chapters when those unchanging relationships are discussed. Chapter 2 then goes on to expose the *evolutionary forces* at work in healthcare by moving through decades-long examples of cause and effect that have shaped today's system.

Finally, Chapter 2 introduces the notion of *compensatory dissonance,* which is what happens in healthcare when dissonance, or discord, in one part of the system leads another part of the system to create further dissonance in compensation. In daily life, we see compensatory dissonance when we try to solve a problem, only to find we have created another, even worse one. Compensatory dissonance is pervasive because the healthcare system has no coordinating infrastructure within which to manage its operations and growth. Each element of the system is remarkably free to go its own way. This lack of discipline and coordination evidenced by compensatory dissonance is a key background concept for understanding the problems with CHINs.

The second key background concept, that of *quality assurance* in clinical care, is the subject of Chapter 3. Concern for quality is positioned as the most important and far-reaching policy issue on the healthcare horizon today. Coverage of quality issues in the context of this book is of major importance because almost every CHIN goal statement includes a commitment to improving quality. The chapter refers to those groups behind the concern for quality and gives the reasons for their concern. It discusses the aspects of quality assurance that have become issues in CHIN development. The chapter focuses on the nature of quality indicators, the difference between enterprise-based and population-based standards of care, and the reasons why these distinctions are critical to the strategies of healthcare executives who are planning for future systems.

Given the conceptual background on goals, stage of evolution, and quality, the subsequent three chapters show healthcare executives how to ensure that the CHIN planning process will meet their enterprise and community goals for the CHIN. Chapter 4 begins by pointing out the great extent to which today's system dissonance is tied up in the *information flow block*. This blockage can take many forms: needed information does not yet exist (e.g., adequate quality indicators); information exists but does not yet flow (e.g., paper-based patient records); or solutions to the dissonance depend substantially on information existing but not yet widely available (e.g., access to more and better clinical guidelines). To illustrate this point, Chapter 4 develops an *information need view* of healthcare that includes the requirements for information on the systemwide, community, and enterprise levels. It then translates many of these requirements at the community level into *incentives* for initiating a CHIN, because, although it is important not to confuse incentives with goals and plans, incentives are still very important components of CHIN development and promotion. Finally, recognizing the common incentives becomes the basis for collaboration with a CHIN.

Chapter 5 explores whether specific incentives have value and relevance to healthcare system and community goals. To make this determination, a *value assessment* tool is introduced to determine whether or not CHIN plans are congruent with goals. First, the incentives identified in Chapter 4 are reexpressed as short-term capabilities that are typical of those selected by many CHINs for early implementation. These are then assessed for their value, in a two-way table, toward healthcare system goals, community goals, and even CHIN goals. Using this method, it is further possible to determine the *relative value* of the various capabilities to CHIN goals.

The value assessment tool can be difficult to use correctly, because advocates of a particular capability may claim that it is relevant to a goal when it is relevant only through a great stretch of the imagination or not at all. In such a case, healthcare executives who are seriously concerned about the long-term viability of their CHIN investment are well advised to look further for proof. The *building block analysis* introduced in Chapter 6 gives added assistance with that determination. It explains both a bottom-up analysis, where known capabilities and goals are compared, and a top-down analysis, where the capabilities a CHIN should initiate are chosen after goals are selected, and they specifically are chosen to meet those goals. The chapter concludes with a discussion of the need to consider many factors in addition to goal relevance when choosing initial capabilities. In particular, it is important to leverage the expensive information technology and other CHIN assets by using each feature many times over to implement multiple capabilities and serve multiple goal-directed purposes.

The value assessment and building block analysis are relatively straightforward tools for setting CHIN initiators in the right direction. Before developing these ideas further in Chapters 9 through 12, however, a review of additional essential background CHIN concepts is presented in Chapters 7 and 8. These chapters explore a number of practical matters important for successful CHIN planning. They also provide basic information necessary for the discussions of the unifying CHIN in Chapter 9.

Chapter 7 first discusses a number of *information-based developments* important for a CHIN, including the electronic patient record; data repositories; master patient index; safeguards for patient privacy; and standards for medical terminology, data exchange, and clinical practice. The chapter then differentiates *information models* for CHINs (i.e., the basic model versus value-added service models).

Chapter 8 addresses tools and options for building a CHIN infrastructure. Among these are a number of *project management guidelines*, such as due diligence and scope control, which are discussed briefly. *Technical topics* include centralized versus distributed technology, telecommunications, and end-to-end security plans. Finally, basic guidelines for using the *Internet and intranets* are given.

Chapter 9 unifies the information in earlier chapters to show how CHIN functions can be leveraged to meet virtually all of a community's health information needs. First, four scenarios representing significant community healthcare needs illustrate the potential breadth of a CHIN's reach into communities. All the key CHIN elements are defined, and their interrelationships are shown, to highlight how CHINs can leverage their resources for further development.

In each case, the CHIN easily enables initiators to complete a project important to community health, one that cannot be achieved without a CHIN. The scenarios also show the commonalities among the diverse CHINs' approaches, thus reinforcing the economic rationale for CHINs designed for multiple purposes. The most important CHIN function then becomes creation of collaborative mechanisms.

The four CHINs are next brought together into the unifying and unified CHIN. The scope of the unified CHIN makes it clear that CHIN advocates may be "underselling" their CHINs when they are seeking early support. By focusing on limiting the resources needed to begin a CHIN, they may be missing the opportunity to promote the full potential of the CHIN—to garner support based on its true value. Finally, the unified CHIN—now viewed as thoroughly integral to the community healthcare infrastructure—is in effect a Community

Health Information System, or CHIS, a system in its own right rather than simply a networking tool.

Chapter 10 envisions the information-based healthcare system of the future. In a fully automated and integrated healthcare system, the information system has become indistinguishable from the healthcare system. In effect, the information system has become the healthcare system, no longer a servant, but part of the heart and soul of the system. In developing this view, the chapter previews the healthcare system envisioned, comparing it with other information-intensive industries. After exploring further developments that ease the way to information-based healthcare, Chapter 10 shows an ever-wider and more extensive information flow as mature CHINs are linked regionally and nationally for common purposes and goals. It shows how, at last, goals for healthcare as a *system* can be met. Most notable among these is the enabling of a healthcare system infrastructure within which the system can plan and manage its affairs.

Chapter 11 discusses the prospects for achieving significant CHINs and makes recommendations on pursuing this goal. The chapter begins by examining complex barriers to the development of CHINs—and eventually CHISs, regional health information systems (RHISs), and national health information systems (NHISs) as well. These barriers exist interdependently at all levels of health care from offices, enterprises, and communities to the system itself and even its social environment, and they range from the technical and organizational to the political and sociological. Finally, the chapter offers recommendations for changing the climate for CHINs. These proposals, directed primarily toward healthcare executives and enterprises, also address the national organizations whose leadership is essential for the collaborative work required to create the healthcare information infrastructure.

References

Community Medical Network (COMNET) Society. 1995. *COMNET's HIN Market Directory, 1996 edition.* Atlanta, GA: Community Medical Network Society.

Duncan, K. A. 1995. "Evolving Community Health Information Networks." *Frontiers of Health Services Management* 12 (1): 5–41.

Hanlon, P. 1994. "CHINs: Lead? Follow? Get Out of the Way?" *Infocare* (November/December): 10.

Hoban, F. T. (ed.). 1995. *Wisconsin Health Information Network: Your Healthcare Connection.* Brookfield, WI: Wisconsin Health Information Network.

John A. Hartford Foundation. 1993. *Annual Report.* 14. New York: John A. Hartford Foundation.

CHAPTER 2

THE EVOLVING
HEALTHCARE SYSTEM

The fortunes of CHINs are bound up in the fortunes of healthcare itself as a system. When a system is in a high state of dissonance, as healthcare surely is today, even essential innovations such as the integration of information technology in CHINs are certain to take second place to institutional and enterprise struggles to survive. The inverse must also be acknowledged, however, since the future of healthcare lies deeply imbedded in the highly symbiotic relationship between healthcare and its information networks (Duncan 1994). In fact, the flow of information, perhaps better characterized as an information "trickle," is a central determinant in many of the unyielding issues in today's healthcare.

Clearly the healthcare system needs CHINs, but several characteristics of the system hamper their development. Understanding these characteristics, and overcoming their negative effects, begins with clarifying the goals of the healthcare system (and thus the goals of CHINs). The next step is to examine certain aspects of the evolution of the modern (post-World War II) healthcare system, by assessing how the system has strayed from the pursuit of its goals and has created the extensive dissonance that affects its ability to function. Finally, the implications of these developments for CHINs are discussed.

ESTABLISHING SYSTEMWIDE GOALS

Chapter 1 discussed the need to set healthcare goals before forming health information networks in general, and CHINs in particular.

13

It also expressed the need for congruence between CHIN objectives and the goals of the system they serve. In dealing with the need for congruence, it is essential to understand first that, in the United States, healthcare has come to be considered as basic and essential a right as food and shelter, rather than as an optional consumer item. Thus, the generally accepted mission for healthcare as a system is to ensure the health of its population. Healthcare goals derive from that mission and are generally believed to be these: **The system should strive to achieve and maintain health for each individual and to provide high-quality healthcare for all who need it, at an affordable price.**

The requirement to set goals applies not only to the system as a whole but also to those subordinate elements of the system (i.e., providers, payors, policymakers) whose mission and actions must be consistent with one or more of the system's goals. The actions of a provider, for instance, must be consistent with health maintenance/improvement, high-quality care, affordability, or all three. A CHIN must in turn support these goals as well.

Congruence of goals heads the list of key properties of successful CHINs. The interrelationships between the goals of different system elements (providers, consumers, payors, etc.) and the ability to launch and sustain successful CHINs are the focus of much of this book. The essential first step in developing congruence of goals, however, is to develop a systemwide perspective of healthcare that will show how the goals of the healthcare system trickle down to influence the success of system elements at all levels.

When we look at the system as a whole, and at the working together of its parts to make a "successful" system, we are using a *systems perspective*. This perspective is a useful tool in interpreting trends and developing extrapolations into the future. Figure 2.1 shows schematically the interrelationship of the healthcare system and its elements, overlaid with health information networks.

The situation of today's healthcare system and its future direction are largely a product of its history in this country and the forces that have shaped its development, rather than of the dissonances so evident today. To foresee where CHINs will be needed, and the incentives that will drive CHIN development, it is necessary to understand those underlying and still active forces.

THE EVOLUTIONARY PATH OF HEALTHCARE

The recent rapid changes in the healthcare system, such as the rush to prepaid care, are generally acknowledged to be part of, or the result of, several significant trends that extend back as far as post–World War II.

Figure 2.1 The Healthcare System and Subsystems Linked by Health Information Networks

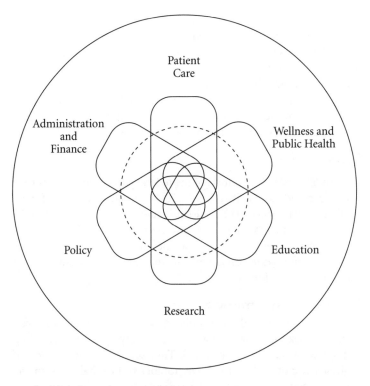

– – – health information network

Many of these trends are directly relevant both to our high need for information networks in healthcare and to our difficulty in creating and using the networks effectively. For instance, the tremendous amount of new medical information derived mainly from newly published research, increasing pressures to contain costs, shifting organizational structures, and rising consumer expectations all have converged to play a key role in healthcare information requirements over the past several decades. The evolutionary path of each of these factors, described in the next sections, is subsequently discussed in terms of their impact on today's healthcare system.

The Post-War Information Explosion

Government funding for medical research increased rapidly after World War II. As professional journals and textbooks proliferated over the next several decades and as experience with modern medicine developed, medical school teaching methods appeared to be unable to keep pace. Dissemination of the new medical information to practicing physicians also lagged, sometimes for years. By the 1980s most observers understood not only that the volume of the factual medical knowledge base of medicine far outstripped the ability of most physicians to keep up with it, but that the system itself did not facilitate the integration of new information with the old to make the medical knowledge base useful to physicians throughout the country. This situation persists today. Further, despite the information glut, much essential medical knowledge is quite remarkable for the gaps that appear in it, as researchers in healthcare quality will attest.

Curbing Costs

The laudable post-War efforts of the federal government to improve healthcare and extend its access quickly turned to concern for its escalating costs (Starr 1982). The subsequent cost-containment policies of governments appear to have been haphazardly conceived, and the consequences of these policies marked the beginning of painful compensatory dissonance in the system. Two examples of the consequences follow.

Healthcare as a market

For several post-War decades policymakers acted on the mistaken belief that healthcare was a market commodity operating according to the laws of supply and demand. They supported the creation of a physician glut and an excessive number of hospital beds, in the expectation that competition for patients would reduce prices per unit of care. They did not consider the possibility that the healthcare system itself would find a more natural way to support this surplus in our then heavily insured, fee-for-service system—by raising the amount of care to be paid for.

The excess physician and bed capacity created its own demand—for more funding to sustain the excess. The bloated healthcare system was ripe for, and welcomed, a force powerful enough to reduce prices on a systemwide basis. After a narrow escape from a federal government takeover of the system in 1993, elements of the system welcomed managed care as a private sector approach that would bring market forces to bear on healthcare costs. The leading edge of healthcare moved from fee-for-service to prepaid care with astonishing speed. The quest for profits in the private sector first cut gross waste from the system and then, emboldened by the shocking lack of professional or organized resistance, cut back on services. The latter is an example of compensatory dissonance that may, in the long run, doom private sector control of healthcare financing.

The Medicare program

The well-intentioned Medicare program of 1965 had benefited millions, but its role as a federal entitlement had also created more mischief than anyone could have foreseen. It was good that millions of aging Americans could now get the healthcare they needed, and thousands of physicians and hospitals conditioned to delivering charity care could now be paid for their services. As a result, however, the total amount of care in the system—and, of course, the total cost of that care—increased dramatically. Healthcare began to be viewed as a right, and physicians began to expect to be paid. The culture of healthcare was changed forever.

When Medicare attempted to curb its own exploding costs in October 1983 through the introduction of prospective payment for diagnosis-related groups (DRGs), it opened the door to the violation of fee-for-service medicine. Perhaps even worse, in terms of dissonance in the system, was that financially pressed inpatient enterprises felt compelled to employ ways of gaming the system: by, for example, upcoding DRGs to a more complex and expensive related diagnosis; and by costshifting, where fee-for-service patients paid part of the cost of treating Medicare patients. Medicine's previous besetting sins had been those of omission and ignorance; now it had added sins of commission. On the positive side, in order to survive with the reduced reimbursement imposed by DRGs, healthcare institutions with a substantial proportion of Medicare patients did begin to use proven management techniques borrowed from other industries in an attempt to reduce their own costs.

Despite clear-cut goals for healthcare as a whole, the predominant pressure on healthcare executives over the past two decades has been to reduce prices. Modern management skills have become the norm, but even good management has failed to contain costs to the satisfaction of purchasers. Thus has the stage been set for introduction of the profit motive. As the primary purchasers of healthcare, large corporations and the federal government, through its Medicare, Medicaid, and employee programs, have been more than ready to let private industry show them how prices could be further reduced.

The Reorganizing System

The shocking speed with which managed care plans such as preferred provider organizations (PPOs) and health maintenance organizations (HMOs) have achieved dominance highlights the rudderless plight of the healthcare system. This wholesale change has affected far more elements of the system than the readily apparent shifts in organization of service delivery and mode of payment. Managed care has also broken down the traditional patterns of academic medicine, clinical research, the healthcare workforce, and physicians' professional stature.

As alliances form, re-form, and even fail, the new enterprises must cope not only with cost containment and new styles of care, but with shifting partners, including new kinds of partners such as home care agencies and disease management organizations; a changing physician population; and a variable patient population—this at a time when every change brings new and unwanted pressures. Managed care plans are being challenged by even newer models for organizing and financing healthcare. Managed competition has a substantial foothold in several states. Medical savings accounts (MSAs), virtual enterprises, and direct contracting with doctors and hospitals in provider-sponsored organizations and physician management organizations are emerging as approaches that challenge the dominance of commercial health plans.

In a healthcare system such as ours, a system seemingly without controls or management, the one certainty is that the organization of service delivery and financing will undergo change again and again. Survivors will be those with a systems perspective, sufficient and appropriate information tools, and the flexibility to meet the challenge with orderly change.

Consumer Expectations

As medicine began to conquer many of its scourges, the majority of people began to view it as something they had to have. Indeed, the fee-for-service healthcare system itself had good reason to encourage that view. Because they were not schooled in medicine and its limitations, and because their own money was not at stake, most consumers never developed a market approach to acquiring healthcare services through careful consideration of need, quality, and cost. Instead, consumers built a satisfying, trusting relationship with their primary physicians and left all decisions to them. This kind of relationship persisted for decades. But it worked against efforts at cost containment, thus expanding the dissonance in the system.

In the past two decades, research into the factors of a healthy life created a new information flow to consumers. At the same time, providers began to make clinical information, as a marketing tool, readily available to patients. Consumers' subsequent rising healthcare sophistication coincided—or collided—with the movement toward prepaid healthcare and its need to cut services in order to contain costs and preserve profits.

Consumers by now were well exposed to a view of medical care that differed from their past assumptions, when they had trusted their physicians and the doctors had made all the decisions. They became increasingly—and perhaps devastatingly for the system—concerned with denial or skimping of services, a lack of prevention and health-building services and concern, and lack of information about the quality of care provided by individual caregivers, institutions, and health plans. Although consumers still were not paying for care, it was clear to them that their care might be substandard—not because full services were too expensive but because profits had to be made from their premiums.

PROGRESS TOWARD SYSTEM GOALS

The high-impact trends just discussed are singularly lacking in relevance to the goals of healthcare and, in some cases, they run counter to the system's goals. Consider these examples.

Access and Quality

None of the identified trends is directed toward improving access to healthcare for all Americans. The number of Americans without insurance is growing steadily. Worth noting especially is the plight of uninsured children.

Although the body of medical knowledge is vast, it is substantially, and to some extent unnecessarily, incomplete. Further, our competence in bringing that knowledge to bear with order and credibility on patients' current or potential problems has not kept pace. As a result, the quality of the healthcare system itself—even beyond quality of care—is rising rapidly to the top of the list of important health system issues.

Affordability

Changes in organization and financing have resulted in temporary cost savings for specific elements of the healthcare system. However, the new payment mechanisms are not those that will lead to a less costly healthcare system. Many experts believe there is ample money in healthcare to take care of everyone's health needs, but achieving this would require reallocation of the healthcare dollar. That is, it is reasonable that savings gained in the system should be devoted to improving the system, by, for example, encouraging the population to adopt healthier lifestyles, putting more emphasis on preventive care and follow-up care, taking advantage of information technology to develop less expensive but more effective styles of healthcare delivery, increasing the relevance of medical education, or improving information flow, or by combining some or all of these improvements. Instead, a substantial part of the savings to provider corporations is being taken out of the system in the form of executive renumeration and profits. One author has likened this practice to "strip mining" the healthcare system (Detmer 1997).

COMPENSATORY DISSONANCE

The healthcare system today is undeniably in a state of dissonance. Many of the most striking new features of the system are not evolutionary in the sense of moving the healthcare system closer to its goals. Rather they are the elements of a painful dissonance that is diverting the system from its goals. Dissonance frequently begins in a system through unintended, and even well-meant, changes. These changes may have been outside the control of the system—for example, a recession—or they may have been intended, like the introduction of Medicare, to serve system goals. The failure to consider the system as a whole—the big picture—has led to partial solutions that negatively affect other parts of the system. Narrow views, often ambiguous or at odds, stand in the way of crafting truly useful solutions to systemwide problems.

When one part of the system creates a dissonance, another part of the system may see a need to compensate for the effect by creating what amounts to further dissonance. This is called *compensatory dissonance*. The evolutionary paths described earlier in this chapter supply several examples of the influence of dissonance on other elements throughout the system. The result is a cascading series of dissonances, each one triggered by the one before and each running increasingly counter to the goals of the system.

- A couple of decades ago, when healthcare costs began increasing rapidly as a share of the gross domestic product, the healthcare system did not act to contain costs. Thus, since it was not acting as a responsible social system it was creating an unacceptable dissonance in American society. Unfortunately, the system as a whole *could not act* because it had no infrastructure within which to set policy and manage its affairs. Powerful key elements of the system, such as physician or hospital organizations, also chose not to band together and act, thus opening the door to outside influence and further dissonance. First the government walked through the door, then the business sector.

- When the Health Care Financing Administration (HCFA) introduced prospective payment to hospitals for Medicare patients, it created considerable dissonance in the fee-for-service system. No system goal was served by this move, but it did turn the entire incentive system and culture of these institutions upside down. The longstanding incentive that led to providing all possible needed care to each patient changed course to become an incentive to care as little as possible for each patient—a compensatory dissonance. Inability to cope with the reversed incentives led to the financial ruin and closure of many hospitals. Since a more complicated diagnosis meant higher payment, many hospitals resorted to upcoding DRGs to ease the financial pressure—a further compensatory dissonance.

- HCFA's cost-cutting success with Medicare's prospective payment for inpatient care led to further experimentation with paying for outpatient care on a fixed-fee schedule. Because HCFA had the power to set these fees, it chose to do so by rewarding primary care with higher fees than in the past and by cutting the fees for certain specialty services. Although this move created dissonance in the physician community, physicians on the whole accepted the change. This act of social engineering was not lost on the for-profit sector, which based its presumption that the physician community would not object to payment manipulation at least in part on this Medicare experiment.

- The for-profit health businesses were the first to move boldly into the hitherto inviolate realm of clinical medicine. Anecdotal evidence of managed care's cuts in expensive patient services shocked Americans, and when business began to skimp wholesale on highly visible services, the dissonance throughout the country became too great to continue without a response. Well-publicized examples of this dissonance were allowing new mothers and their babies only one day of observation and care after delivery, and sending mastectomy patients home after one day. So the backlash began. Because the physician community had tolerated this commercial interference in doctor-patient relationships, Congress felt it had to step in to protect patients from both their provider organizations and their physicians. When Congress provided legislative relief for the new mothers and babies and the mastectomy patients, it created a compensatory dissonance with far-reaching implications for government interference in the practice of medicine. Again, physicians on the whole did not object. They allowed clinical care practices to be legislated and revealed themselves collectively to be powerless in the face of whatever forces were likely to sweep over the healthcare system.

Dissonances and compensatory dissonances abound in for-profit healthcare. While managed care has much to offer the beleaguered healthcare system, those who employ managed care are using it in ways that invite countermeasures. These include not only cutting patient services to avoid costs but also selecting healthier enrollees and opting not to pay their fair share for medical education and research. These in turn create further dissonance in the system and inevitably lead to such artificialities as risk adjustment and piecemeal legislation.

Dissonance is expensive and destructive. When elements in a system are engaged in escalating dissonance, they are not moving toward goals either for themselves or the system. All of the examples of compensatory dissonance in this section run counter to system goals and have hampered our progress toward an optimally healthy society. When physicians individually and collectively fail to act in the best interests of their patients, and when hundreds of billions of dollars can easily and legally be diverted from the medical care for which it is intended, the system is out of control.

Dissonance in the healthcare system carries over into CHIN development efforts as well. It emerges early in the planning stages in the conflicting goals and contradictory incentives at work in the community and especially among CHIN participants. A case in point is the clash of differing views about whether or not information heretofore considered proprietary should be shared through a CHIN. For instance, purchasers and consumer groups want providers to make available information on quality of care in their enterprises so that the community stakeholders can make informed selections of providers. But providers do not want to make this information available in their communities because of its potential usefulness to their competitors and the possibility that non-healthcare professionals might misinterpret or misuse the information. Dissonance in the CHIN escalates when the purchasers and consumer groups' goals are adopted but goal implementation remains in the hands of the provider groups with a different agenda.

The most significant implication of the current system dissonance is a new—some say overdue—focus on assuring the quality of medical care. The reach of this development will touch every aspect of healthcare, especially acute and chronic patient care, medical education, and clinical research. The coming quality revolution is the subject of the next chapter, which provides background for discussing the extensive and essential role for CHINs in quality assurance.

References

Detmer, D. E. 1997. "The Future of the IAIMS in a Managed Care Environment: A Call for Private Action and Public Investment."

Journal of the American Medical Informatics Association 4 (2): Supplement 65–71.

Duncan, K. A. 1994. *Health Information and Health Reform: Understanding the Need for a National Health Information System.* San Francisco: Jossey-Bass.

Starr, P. 1982. *The Social Transformation of American Medicine.* New York: Basic Books.

CHAPTER 3

THE COMING QUALITY REVOLUTION

T he primary legacy of dissonance in any system is the erosion of quality, and this is certainly the perception in healthcare. Consumers, purchasers, accreditors, and policymakers are demanding information about quality because they intend to demand quality. For providers, participation in quality assurance processes today is not an option. In fact, issues surrounding quality assurance are leading to the biggest revolution in healthcare since the Flexner Report in 1910 forever changed the process of medical education (Starr 1982).

Quality is a far-reaching issue that involves all aspects of the healthcare system, including not just clinical care and service but also the processes of clinical research, professional education, policy formation, and planning. However, it is clear that, as practitioners of care and custodians of patient records, providers and payors hold the keys to quality healthcare because they are the people in a position to assess and improve care (Eddy 1996). Thus, for healthcare executives, quality of care will continue to be a growing concern for which it will be shown that cooperative use of the tools of information technology—such as CHIN development—is indispensable.

As quality of care moves to the top of the research and policy agenda, it may well become the driving force behind new cooperatively initiated health information networks. In fact, most CHINs have improvement in the quality of care as an explicit goal. The belief that CHINs can improve quality, especially through administrative measures, is pervasive, attracting the participation of many non-healthcare players such as banks, vendors, and systems houses, and even technology-challenged physicians. But one needs to describe improvement in quality and to specify how a CHIN can become a quality improvement mechanism.

Healthcare executives need to understand the scope and importance of the quality debate as an information issue, in order to give quality its appropriate priority in selecting among information technology options. This chapter explores several dimensions of the quality issue, to provide further background for discussions about CHIN success factors.

STAKEHOLDERS IN QUALITY ASSURANCE

Quality assurance has two major components, quality assessment and quality acquisition. *Quality assessment* measures the existing level of quality anywhere in the healthcare system, but especially in patient care. *Quality acquisition* comprises those measures used to raise the level of quality higher than it has been assessed to be.

Consumers are deeply concerned about the quality of healthcare they can get from their health plans. However, a recent national survey showed that consumers today are forced to use primarily nonquality-related factors in selecting a health plan, because good quality measures simply are not available to them (Robinson and Brodie 1997).

Consumers' time-honored ways of assessing quality have been licensure for physicians and accreditation for hospitals. This rather far-removed evidence of adequate professional competence was convincing in the past when patients trusted their physicians and nurses to do their best. Today, however, several factors have converged to erode that trust. A growing volume of evidence shows extensive variability among important parameters of care given by physicians and other providers. Even more unnerving are the stories about health plans withholding care for seriously ill patients, which consumers are reading or hearing about almost daily in newspapers and magazines and on television. Most distressing is the perception that community physicians who participate in plans have been unwilling or unable to protect their managed care patients from cost-cutting administrators.

As the perception of quality of care erosion becomes more widespread, consumers want more and better information on quality. They want that information to be meaningful, easy to understand, and easy to use as a basis for selecting among plans and providers. But consumers are just one of six significant groups determined to acquire information on quality.

A second group comprises the purchasers, primarily employers and governments. This group wants to understand the rationale and implications of plan pricing, but members also want to know that they are choosing or offering healthcare coverage of known good quality. In fact, those who purchase healthcare for others, such as pension plans, have a fiduciary responsibility for the quality of that care (Greenfield 1996). Because purchasers need proof that health plans are delivering care as promised, they will continue to demand more and better information about quality of care.

The third group is made up of those who accredit healthcare organizations and license facilities and professionals. These are the bodies to whom both payors and consumers currently look as the best sources of information on quality, even though these organizations measure quality far from adequately. If they are to retain their positions as arbiters of quality, accreditors and licensors must be able to collect, analyze, and present increasingly sophisticated ratings (Rulon 1996).

The fourth group is policymakers at all levels of government, foundations, and professional organizations. Each has constituencies, missions, and concerns for assuring and improving the quality of healthcare.

The fifth group, the payors, includes insurance companies and healthcare plans such as HMOs that want to be certain they are paying only for necessary care.

The sixth group comprises providers and other healthcare delivery enterprises wanting to be certain that the care they provide or arrange meets the highest possible standards. In the quality equation their position is unique because they have the major responsibility for meeting the quality information needs of the remaining stakeholders as well as their own.

Whether quality information is being provided for consumers, providers, purchasers, payors, policymakers, or accreditors, all but the most rudimentary information is very expensive and laborious to collect after the care is given. For instance, in 1996 a California health plan coalition paid $1 million for its 25 members to be evaluated on just six preventive services (Kertesz 1996). The effectiveness of many preventive services is questionable, and in any case they certainly are not indicators of the general or specific quality of a healthcare plan's activities. With the relatively primitive methods currently used to measure quality, it is much easier for a health plan to game the quality measures by making improvements in the areas they measure than it is to come to grips with the quality issue as a whole.

Because of the information-intensive nature of quality assurance in any form, it merits serious consideration in any discussion of health information networks. In fact, the quest for quality of care may well be the primary driving force and incentive for forming future health information networks, especially CHINs.

QUALITY IN HEALTHCARE

What is behind the quality of care debate, and why has it recently become such a visible issue? Just where does our health system stand in terms of achieving a reasonable quality? How is quality defined, and how can it be improved? These questions are the next subject for discussion.

Why Quality of Care?

Why is the issue of quality healthcare so difficult? First of all, it is a distasteful issue in that demanding proof of quality is indicative of a troubling lack of trust in our healthcare professionals and in-stitutions. In turn, many distrustful providers hesitate to provide information about their performance, because they believe it may be misinterpreted or misunderstood by purchasers and the public. It is the public's past unquestioned trust in America's healthcare teams that has brought about the current dilemma relating to quality of care. That complacency has led to a massive and complex healthcare system that, unthinkably, holds the health and lives of millions in its control without a system of quality control.

Although consumers and purchasers want high-quality care, it is reasonable for providers to hesitate to guarantee it. This is because neither purchasers, consumers, nor any other groups directly involved in the healthcare system really know how to go about getting quality information. None of us truly can define the quality of healthcare that can be achieved, how to measure it, or how to change practice patterns individually or systematically when quality is not what it should be. Further, many professionals believe that the best approach to ensuring quality care is through education and guidance *before or at the moment of care*, rather than checking after the fact to see if quality care was delivered. These various issues are discussed more extensively in later sections of this chapter.

Can Quality of Care Be Defined?

Little consensus has been reached on what constitutes quality health-care. For instance, extensive research dating back at least ten years shows that in comparable situations, some medical procedures are performed notably more often in some locations than in others (Wennberg 1987). Such a variation in incidence ("practice variation") surely is not acceptable, at least to patients, but the impact to date of such research on clinical practice patterns has been minimal.

Practice variation is an example of perhaps the most compelling of several quality dimensions: provider competence. Other key dimensions of quality include health plan competence and health system competence. Each is discussed next, from a consumer perspective, to illustrate the breadth of the concerns that the providers supplying the quality information will need to address.

Provider competence

The dimension of provider competence encompasses a range of parameters including at least basic intelligence, motivation, and ethics; medical education; continuing medical education; problem solving skills; interpersonal skills; and appropriateness of settings and tools. Typical questions of interest are these:

- Is there more to be known about my problem than my doctor knows?
- How can I be sure my doctor is considering the latest and most complete information?
- How do I know my doctor is considering only my best interests?
- How do I know if my doctor is completely frank with me?
- Do any of the doctors available to me know all there is to know about my problem or how to find out?
- Which doctors are most skilled at doing this procedure?
- Is my hospital team skilled at dealing with my problem?
- How can I find out this information?

Health plan competence

The dimension of health plan competence includes at least the parameters of services, value, commitment to the individual, commitment to provider excellence, and appropriate use of such tools of disease management as consumer and patient education, preventive care, follow-up, and home care. These are the quality-related questions that might be asked here:

- Is competent advice available at all times?
- Is medical care available at all times?
- Are the professionals employed by the plan among the best in their fields?
- May I see the type of health professional I believe I need to see?
- May I select and see the same physician regularly?
- Does my physician have complete freedom to exercise the best clinical judgment on my behalf?

- What treatment choices do I have, and what is the process for choosing?
- Are processes for obtaining care clear and easy to follow?
- What happens if I do not agree with the plan on any matter?
- How well does the plan take care of members who are sick?
- Does my plan pay for experimental therapies?
- How well does the plan catch health problems in the early stages?
- What can I do for myself to stay healthy?
- What can I do for myself to avoid seeing a doctor unnecessarily?
- What can I do to take care of my chronic problem myself?
- What preventive care services are available?
- What preventive care services are valuable?
- Where can I get up-to-date medical information?
- Are the facilities pleasant, convenient, and easy to use?
- Does my plan offer me multiple communication channels?

Health system competence

Issues in health system competence go far beyond the ability of an individual or group to get competent medical care. Health system competence begins, once again, with consideration of the mission and goals of the system. Questions center on whether or not the system is doing what it can and should do to achieve and maintain good health for all, including the provision of high-quality care at an affordable price. As its top priority the system as a whole should be concerned with the ability of all Americans to get the medical care they need. Related issues include the quality of medical education, the amount and appropriateness of medical research, the flow of information to those who want and need it throughout the system, the formation of policy and of planning structures for future needs, and the coordination and management of all elements of the system. Consumer questions might typically be these:

- Does anyone besides me have this problem?
- Is anyone doing research on this problem?
- How do I find out what is known or being studied?
- How and when does my doctor find new information?
- How might the results of current research affect me?
- So many people are not able to get the medical care they need: What are the real reasons? Is anyone collecting information or studying why?
- How can I avoid becoming one of these people?
- This is such a rich country: Why can my family not get the medical care it needs?

- Are there not easier, cheaper ways to get medical care than going to see a doctor?
- Are doctors today being taught more about nutrition, prevention, and alternative approaches to care than they used to be?
- On whom do medical students, interns, and residents practice? Who pays them?
- What is the state of the art in nutrition and wellness?
- Where do I go for nutrition and wellness information?
- Who decides how many doctors and hospitals we need?
- Who is responsible for public health, and what are they doing?
- Who is doing studies on costs, and what happens to the money that is saved?
- Who, if anyone, makes systemwide decisions about healthcare?

Questions asked by purchasers, accreditors, policymakers, and planners cover the same range of parameters, but with many additional, highly significant concerns already well known to healthcare executives. These include administrative parameters such as cost, availability of resources, and program effectiveness. The concerns of these latter four groups are also legitimate and must be addressed.

How Can Quality be Measured?

As the medical knowledge base grows and becomes more complete and sophisticated, standards of quality should evolve to keep pace. Even if a consensus exists on what quality of care means today, we still are faced with the difficulty of measuring it. Part of the problem is a lack of available comparable data across institutions. The only consistently collected data are those collected by insurance companies for payment purposes, and these data reveal little beyond diagnoses and treatments. Any other studies of the kind of care, individual or collective, being given at an institution would most likely require a laborious search through individual medical records. The quality of the raw data in medical records is also questionable, as the traditional view of health professionals is that record keeping is a chore of secondary importance to patient care. Several other issues relating to measuring quality, while not necessarily more important, are at least as complex as these and merit a separate discussion later in this section. Some of these issues are:

- the use of surrogate versus direct indicators of quality;
- prospective quality assurance (implemented before or at the time of care) versus retrospective quality assurance (measured after the time of care); and
- enterprise versus population standards of care.

Can Quality Be Improved?

Quality experts agree that we are capable of a much higher standard of care than is routinely available. For instance, although the healthcare system received with great interest the information on practice variation noted earlier, little was—or could be—done about the problem. This situation highlights yet another quality problem— the *information block*, noted in Chapter 1, that is a result of the scarcity of channels for information in healthcare. Put another way, even though a systematic quality problem such as practice variation may become widely known, the healthcare system does not have an adequate mechanism for translating that knowledge into a measurable impact on clinical practice patterns. Physicians on the whole simply do not or cannot assimilate and integrate the new information so that their patients can benefit from it. In the case of practice variation, for instance, individual physicians who have the time and resources might compare their own rates to the norm for a particular procedure such as cesarean deliveries and consider making changes in their own practices. They may even be urged to do so by their county, state, or national specialty societies. But what the system actually needs are practical and routinely available mechanisms for integrating and using new and valuable information like this, whenever and wherever it becomes known, to modify clinical practices.

In a further example of the information block, in so many areas of medicine not enough is known about the causes and courses of diseases, or the effects of various therapies, such that standards for high-quality care could be established. Much more could be known if, in some orderly manner, we could tap the billions of pieces of information in the file folders containing patient records. Surprisingly, records of the experiences of all patients who are being treated in hospitals and clinics are scarcely used at all to improve medical knowledge about the best approaches to care. And worse, much of what we do know lies buried and virtually inaccessible in the millions of research articles that have appeared through the years in thousands of medical journals and textbooks.

Clearly, good information is the key to quality improvement throughout the system. Consider the case of quality improvement of clinical care. On the one hand, current medical knowledge needs to flow to physicians and other providers in a form that is useful and timely. Just as essential, however, is that specific patient information flow back from providers, through clinical researchers for analysis and integration, and into the knowledge base. Figure 3.1 shows this synergistic information cycle. It serves as a reminder that access to information about current patient experience is a key to keeping the medical knowledge base (MKB) as current as possible.

Figure 3.1 The Clinical Information Quality Cycle

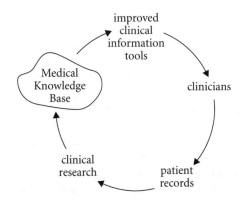

The information flow for quality improvement of health services is similar. Health plans must collect information about their services for health services researchers to add to that body of knowledge. In turn, health plans can draw on that collective body of knowledge to improve services. Without these critical information flows, it is hard to see how quality can be positively affected except within relatively small pockets of the system.

ISSUES IN MEASURING QUALITY OF CARE

Definitions of quality, deciding what to measure and how to measure it, and the expense and difficulty of obtaining reliable data are among the practical issues to be tackled in quality assurance. The issues selected here for discussion, however, are concepts that underlie the more practical problems; they deal with the nature of indicators (measures) of quality, two different, complementary approaches to implementing quality, and an issue that highlights the need for cooperative development of quality assurance approaches.

In each case, current approaches to measuring quality are simplistic and will be seen as inadequate. The practice of quality assurance is certain to grow more complex. Healthcare executives need to understand and consider these concepts as a part of the quality assurance framework within which the more practical problems are addressed.

The Nature of Quality Indicators

Not all so-called indicators of quality in use today serve any real purpose. This section considers primarily the misuse of surrogate indicators of the quality of clinical care. Surrogate indicators are those in which something that is relatively easy to measure is taken as an indicator of the quality of something that is difficult to measure. For instance, an accrediting body might want to know the rate of surgical complications at a hospital or within a health plan, but finding this information in the medical records of all surgery patients needed to answer this question would be virtually impossible. Instead, the complication rate of a single type of surgery such as carotid endarterectomy is used as an *indicator* of the relative acceptability of the complication rates for all surgeries at that hospital.

While the surrogate indicator approach to assessing quality may be less than ideal, it does seem to be a practical approach that many evaluators have adopted for the time being. Besides the questionable inherent value of surrogate indicators, there is at least one other problem. Since the particular surgery or procedure being used as a surrogate is usually known in advance, it is relatively straightforward to ensure that all surgeries or preventive measures of that type are conducted with great care, thus assuring a high "score." This kind of approach is another instance of gaming the system.

An even less satisfactory practice is the use of surrogate indicators such as immunization rates, cervical cancer screening, or selected outpatient procedures to assess quality of care for plans that also treat serious illnesses. This is the approach taken by the National Committee for Quality Assurance (NCQA), the leading accreditor of managed care plans, in the latest version of its Health Plan Employer Data and Information Set (HEDIS) (Iglehart 1996). A prospective member of the plan might prefer to know more about the completeness of care given to patients who, for example, are seriously ill with cancer or chronically ill with asthma or diabetes.

The most suspect of surrogate indicators is patient satisfaction with clinical care. While it is certainly important that patients be satisfied with their care, they may be the last to know when their outcomes are suboptimal or that the processes used in diagnosing and treating their problems are not the most appropriate. Patients are not the right people to ask.

When they elect to use surrogate measures, the NCQA and other quality-measuring groups, such as the Joint Commission on Accreditation of Healthcare Organizations (JCAHO), and medical groups such as the California Medical Association, are grappling with a very difficult problem, but it is clear that they have not yet gone far enough in requiring appropriate measures.

The tools and methodology exist to identify and use more appropriate quality indicators and measure them (Greenfield et al. 1996; Brook, Kamberg, and McGlynn 1996; Brook, McGlynn, and Cleary

1996). Sophisticated methods of design, analysis, and synthesis, when combined with available information technology, make it possible to create a system of quality assurance of value to the entire healthcare system, including individual enterprises and providers. Although much work lies ahead, today's extensive use of inappropriate surrogate indicators should soon no longer be acceptable.

Prospective versus Retrospective Quality Assurance

Approaches to quality can be prospective or retrospective, and in fact both approaches are essential to a complete *quality assurance system*. Prospective approaches, or *quality acquisition*, are those that are put in place prior to the time of care. Retrospective approaches, or *quality assessment*, are those that measure quality of care after the fact. Each is appropriate in different circumstances, but healthcare executives must ensure that both approaches are implemented at every plan and provider enterprise. That is, the quality assurance equation must be complete:

Quality Assurance = Quality Acquisition + Quality Assessment

Quality acquisition

Prospective approaches to assuring quality include development of medical models that help us understand disease processes; improvment of the medical knowledge base; provision of relevant professional education; careful licensure, certification, or accreditation with periodic reexamination; and ready availability of information for professionals in such forms as reviews, syntheses, databases, expert systems, or clinical guidelines (highly specific advice such as "critical paths"). For prospective quality assurance to affect patterns of care, the information must be extensive, comprehensive, reliable, timely, easy to use and understand, and accessible at the place of service as well as for study.

Many elements of prospective quality assurance, such as education and licensure, are already in place, but more work needs to be done, and providers of care hold the key. To cut costs, providers have been decreasing their organizations' traditional involvement in and responsibility for professional education, research, and other infrastructural concerns. That is, enterprises sensitive to market forces are no longer willing to act as teaching institutions or to support academic medical centers, and they no longer encourage their staffs to engage in clinical research. This trend is unfortunate; the most valuable educational experiences for health professionals occur at the point of care, and the most useful clinical research data flow from actual patient experiences. Thus the participation of most providers in systems of education and research is essential to the continued vitality of healthcare. Similarly, prospective provision for quality care is possible only with the cooperation of providers who collaborate in creating a prospective quality assurance system. They must not only provide data for the ongoing clinical research needed to fuel such a system (Bero and Drummond 1995); they must also use the products of such a system to maintain quality at their institutions. These products would include educational materials at all levels; tools for recertification; guidelines for diagnosis, treatment, and management of disease; and access to expert opinion. Figure 3.2 shows the cycle of dependency between providers and prospective quality assurance.

Quality assessment

Retrospective approaches attempt to measure the quality of care after the care has been given. Among the current standard approaches, which probably include the use of surrogate measures, are (Brook, Kamberg, and McGlynn 1996)

- outcome measurement, of the extent of the patient's ability to return to normal life;
- process measurement, of the appropriateness of the steps taken in the patient's care;
- service measurement, of the patient's perceptions about care;
- explicit adherence to an a priori standard for, for instance, surgical competence; and
- expert opinion, such as peer review.

Figure 3.2   Quality Acquisition: Prospective Quality Assurance

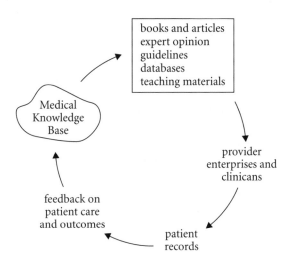

A most important newcomer should be added to this list— a review of the information an enterprise makes available to its caregivers and of how those caregivers use the information. It seems reasonable that a physician with available information resources, who makes extensive use of those educational materials, journals, databases, guidelines, consultations, and expert opinion, is probably practicing better medicine than a physician who does not read, conduct research on behalf of his or her patients, or consult with recognized experts.

Without quality assessment, the knowledge that quality needs to be improved and the incentives to do so are lacking. With quality assessment, the information gleaned is a powerful change agent for actual clinical care. The knowledge gained motivates enterprises, institutions, and providers to modify attitudes and processes, and it triggers a reassessment of the standards of care currently in vogue. Thus quality assessment information has value not only for the providers and enterprises who collect the information, but also for the community and the healthcare system as a whole. Figure 3.3 shows the feedback loop whereby the retrospective measures of quality have multiple effects within healthcare, including their use in helping to upgrade and maintain prospectively established standards of care, as well as in providing needed quality information to consumers, purchases, payors, and providers.

Clearly, prospective and retrospective approaches to quality assurance are equally valuable aspects of the quality solution. Both also have in common a high level of complexity, difficulty, and expense, and both require a corporate and a cultural commitment to the

Figure 3.3   Quality Assessment: Retrospective Quality Assurance

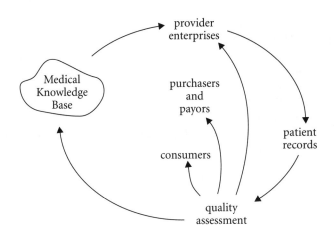

importance of information and quality. For provider enterprises, neither is optional. Consumers, purchasers, accreditors, and policymakers are demanding information about quality because they intend to have quality healthcare.

The quality solution

In planning for quality, healthcare executives should keep in mind that the prospective and retrospective approaches to quality, together with the raw clinical data made available by providers for clinical research, constitute the necessary quality assurance system. Figure 3.4 illustrates the principle that providers need to make patient data available for clinical research and for the development of medical models. These in turn would fuel the development of high-quality professional education, continuing educational materials, databases, and guidelines for use by professionals. To complete the feedback loop, further patient data would be used to assess quality retrospectively in order to motivate institutional change and to continue improving the information tools available to professionals.

Enterprise-Based versus Population-Based Standards

Enterprise-based standards of care rely on past clinical experiences of patients within an enterprise to set treatment policies for future patient care. Healthcare executives need to understand the pitfalls of developing and using these kinds of standards; they should instead rely most heavily on population-based standards that are derived from information on large patient populations and are generally accepted throughout the healthcare system. Population-based standards may be modified by local conditions (such as environmental factors or religious beliefs not pertinent to other areas) into community-based standards for all community providers. Both concepts are now discussed more fully.

Enterprise-based standards

Many providers, especially large physician groups or health plans, are using their own patients' experiences and outcomes to develop quality measures and guidelines for future clinical practice. Standards of care that are developed from information available only to the group or plan are called *enterprise-based standards*. For instance, a physician group might research all available information about managing asthma patients and, combined with studying how their own patients fared under various disease management approaches, they might develop a protocol, or guideline, for the care of asthma patients. Such a guideline would be quite rigorous, specifying hundreds of steps and options to be considered or used, depending on the patient's

Figure 3.4 The Quality Solution

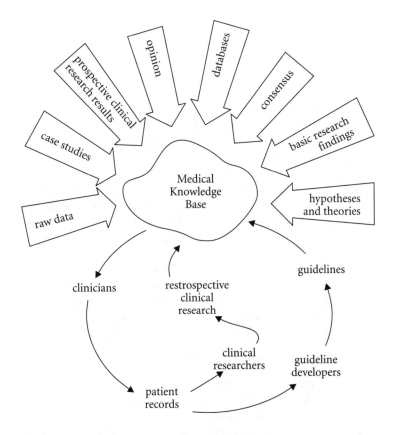

circumstances. In a second example, a health plan might review its own patient population to determine which of two drug regimens or surgical alternatives has worked best at their institutions, and then recommend or require that physicians use the selected option.

It is easy to see that if the sample of patients being considered is relatively small, if the patient population for the period under review was in any way atypical, or if the standards of care are not already high, then the value of the new enterprise-specific standards is questionable. Because of these inherent limitations, any recommendations based on such samples might not be acceptable elsewhere in the community or country. In fact, Wennberg's studies on practice variation have shown us that this situation is likely to be the case. Even when outside information is added to enterprise information, as in the case of the physician group example, busy doctors are unlikely to be able to create and keep updated all of the guidelines they will need in their practices. Thus healthcare executives should be aware that enterprise-based standards for care, especially in complex medical situations, are almost always less than satisfactory.

Population-based standards

Population-based standards of care, on the other hand, use data from large, representative groups throughout the community, region, state, or country. In this case, information from the entire population under consideration is integrated to minimize the biases inherent in dealing only with data from small groups. Guidelines, databases, and other forms of advice and information developed from population-based standards have much broader applicability. Such resources also include information about rare medical problems, complex medical problems, or both. Enterprises that develop their own standards typically do not have enough patients with rare or complex problems to set applicable standards for diagnosing and treating those problems.

Population-based standards have the further advantage of spreading the work of development and maintenance over a much larger group of professionals. By using population-based standards, with community-based modifications, enterprises avoid the almost overwhelming and certainly redundant commitment of resources that would occur if every enterprise were to develop its own guidelines without benefit of ongoing population-level analyses.

THE LAST WORD ON QUALITY

Some of the important quality issues discussed here are already beginning to confront healthcare executives. Quality of healthcare has several powerful stakeholders that will force it to the top of priorities for healthcare system change. It should be apparent that responding to stakeholder concerns will require the extensive use of health information networks. Attention to the issues related to quality measurement is essential to the success of quality solutions that will be based in the health information networks of the future, including CHINs.

Robust but flexible approaches to quality assessment, then, are the key to successful systems. Healthcare executives must plan for advances in quality evaluation theory, practice, and technology, and must be able to adapt to them, as they develop. The competitive advantage will go to those players who have planned well and can easily accommodate new demands.

References

Bero, L., and R. Drummond. 1995. "The Cochrane Collaboration." *Journal of the American Medical Association* 274 (24): 1935–38.

Brook, R. H., C. F. Kamberg, and E. A. McGlynn. 1996. "Health System Reform and Quality." *Journal of the American Medical Association* 276 (6): 476–80.

Brook, R. H., E. A. McGlynn, and P. D. Cleary. 1996. "Quality of Health Care Part 2: Measuring Quality of Care." *The New England Journal of Medicine* 335 (13): 966–70.

Eddy, D. M. 1996. *Clinical Decision Making: From Theory to Practice.* Sudbury, MA: Jones and Bartlett Publishers.

Greenfield, L., B. D. Colen, P. D. Cleary, and S. Greenfield. 1996. *Evaluating the Quality of Health Care: What Research Offers Decision Makers.* New York: Milbank Memorial Fund.

Iglehart, J. K. 1996. "Health Policy Report: The National Committee for Quality Assurance." *The New England Journal of Medicine* 335 (13): 995–98.

Kertesz, L. 1996. "California Report Card Uses Uniform Data." *Modern Healthcare* 26 (25): 102.

Robinson, S., and M. Brodie. 1997. "Understanding the Quality Challenge for Consumers: The Kaiser/AHCPR Survey." *Journal on Quality Improvement* 23 (5): 239–44.

Rulon, V. 1996. "Measurement Systems Beyond HEDIS: The Evolution of Healthcare Data Analysis in Managed Care." *Journal of the American Healthcare Information Management Association* 67 (2): 48–52.

Starr, P. 1982. *The Social Transformation of American Medicine.* New York: Basic Books.

Wennberg, J. E. 1987. "Are Hospital Services Rationed in New Haven or Over-Utilized in Boston?" *Lancet* (May 23): 1185–88.

CHAPTER 4

INFORMATION NEEDS
AND INCENTIVES

The previous chapter makes clear that information is the lifeblood of high-quality medical practice. Part of that essential information is in the form of patient records, and part of it resides in the vast virtual dynamic of a *medical knowledge base* made up of books, journals, databases, research findings, and human thought. The information, which may be memorized or may be accessible with varying degrees of difficulty, is useful only if it is free to flow to the right location in the system when it is needed. Thus, *information flow* is the vital functional infrastructure that makes information useful for medical practice within the enterprise and throughout the system.

The earlier chapter on the evolutionary path of healthcare shows that an amazingly high proportion of the pressures, problems, and needs throughout the healthcare system, in addition to clinical care, are information based. They are the result of either (1) a lack of good information; (2) the failure of available information to flow; or (3) the need for a new information flow for their solution.

This chapter continues to demonstrate the extensive role for CHINs and other health information networks (HINS), first, by translating the pressures on the system into a set of *information needs* that are critical to healthcare at several levels, including the systemwide level, the community level, and the enterprise and provider levels. The final sections of the chapter reframe these needs in terms of the *incentives* that enterprise healthcare executives have for collaborating in meeting those needs. The case is made that the system's successful future depends on cooperative information flow among healthcare enterprises. It is only by recognizing these mutual needs, and the need for mutual solutions, that successful CHINs can be conceived and implemented.

THE INFORMATION-NEED VIEW

The difference between what is good for the healthcare system as a whole and the amount of that "good" that the nation's health plans and providers can reasonably be expected to provide constitutes a vast gulf. Certainly infrastructural issues such as the reform of medical education or support for clinical research and policy formation are beyond the scope of individual enterprises. Further, individual plans and providers/provider groups cannot be expected to solve the problems of access for all Americans, nor can they do much individually to reduce the expense of healthcare except at their own institutions. Nor can enterprises individually address quality as an issue today, when most performance measures are used primarily to compare one enterprise with another. Thus, it seems clear that virtually all progress to be made in the overall healthcare system depends on cooperative action; healthcare executives must step beyond the boundaries of their enterprises to seek common solutions.

The entire healthcare system, from policy and planning to research, teaching, and quality assurance, is structured solely to empower providers and enable them to care for patients and look after the health of the nation. Because the system needs to check its progress, feedback loops are key components for success; that is, if the healthcare system is to function well, participation and feedback from provider enterprises is critical. No other element in healthcare can supply that feedback, because providers at the front line of healthcare are the custodians of the information. Without their cooperation in supplying that information outside the enterprise, healthcare will fail to achieve its potential for excellence.

Although information needs can be viewed in many dimensions, it seems useful at this point to consider them according to whose information needs they are. This will facilitate the later consideration of the incentives enterprises have to meet those various needs.

Healthcare System Needs

The healthcare system needs to meet its goals of access, quality, and affordability. To do so, it needs to create an infrastructure that it does not now have. Because of its complexity, the system needs an orderly way to pull together its diverse elements to focus on goals.

The system needs a way to make policy, survey needs, plan goal-directed programs, conduct prioritized research, offer appropriate educational opportunities, and implement public health programs. It also needs the ability to coordinate, administer, and manage all of these functions and a host of others. In short, it needs an infrastructure within which the essential mission-directed functions of the system can be carried out. The information flow required to achieve such an infrastructure is tremendous, but with the cooperative use of information technology, it can alleviate several of the health system problems identified in earlier chapters. At a minimum the infrastructure should

- relieve the information block and allow new medical information to flow;
- eliminate the need for precipitous organizational change and haphazard cost-containment measures by facilitating meaningful research on the organization and financing of healthcare;
- reassure consumers and purchasers with appropriate quality assurance measures;
- enable researchers to examine ways of solving the problem of access for all;
- use essential feedback from health plans and providers for continuous system improvement; and
- update and maintain the dynamic medical knowledge base.

Needs Common to All Enterprises

All system elements that are concerned with patient care have certain common needs that they cannot meet by themselves. They need to be certain that the resources they require, such as professional staff, capital for improvements, and reliable equipment and supplies, will be available. They need commonly agreed-upon ways to finance the care they deliver. They need continuing education programs and expert-based guidelines for their professional staff members. They need accreditation for their institutions and recertification of professionals. Finally, they need a marketplace within which to compete for patients.

As the system grows steadily in complexity, current approaches to assuring that these needs are met are beginning to fail. Failure to plan and manage the system has led to a physician surplus and a specialty and geographic maldistribution whereby a substantial proportion of the population is underserved. The healthcare financing system is far behind most other information-intensive industries in its adoption of industry standards and information technology. Medical education is moving away from its relevance to society's healthcare needs, and substantive continuing education opportunities are hard to find or take advantage of. The need for better professional information resources such as guidelines has long been evident, but progress toward a useful system of guideline development and dissemination is minuscule when compared to need. By and large, accreditors are unable to obtain meaningful quality assessment for the enterprises they need to accredit. The marketplace is the most uncertain element of all, as the advent of new ways to organize and finance care seems almost to resemble a free-for-all.

The direction of change in each of these arenas is not positive. Healthcare enterprises would be correct in believing that their futures are uncertain in ways that are beyond their individual control. Those that want to survive and thrive into the next century need to join together in seeking common solutions to these problems.

Community-Specific Needs

Healthcare executives know that, whatever organizational format their enterprises enjoy now, they could be very different in two, three, or five years. Their competitors today could be their partners tomorrow, or vice versa: hospitals and doctor groups affiliated today could be competitors tomorrow. Even apparently stable large, for-profit enterprises may break up when profits are no longer available to their shareholders. Each new affiliation requires the creation of new information pathways, and each abandoned one requires that those pathways disentangle. However, if community enterprises were to agree on a common approach to information flow, such as a CHIN can provide, then communication links could easily be established or discontinued, and shifting affiliations and alliances would be spared the major headache of reconfiguring their information systems.

To understand how the CHIN would accomplish this, consider that, in concept, a CHIN is like a phone system. Everyone, whether partner, competitor, or customer, would be connected at all times to the same central network, but only those wishing to communicate with each other would do so. No physical rewiring or new systems designs would be needed when affiliations within a community changed.

Similarly, the population of doctors who contract with specific health plans or who are on the staff of a particular hospital is constantly shifting. Yet physicians need to be in regular communication with plans from the first day of affiliation for such purposes as determining eligibility and guidelines, obtaining pre-approvals, returning statistical information, and obtaining payment. Correspondingly, hospitals are forging electronic links with the offices and homes of their medical staff for such purposes as admitting patients, placing orders, reporting results, and reviewing portions of a patient's medical record. If all community physicians were linked to a common information network, the task of adding physicians to an enterprise's communications link, or removing them from it, would be trivial.

Patient populations shift as well. The concept behind HMOs is that the payment system gives HMOs the incentive to help its members stay as healthy as possible. But it is difficult to find value in developing a healthy member population when members are free to transfer to some other health plan that then becomes the beneficiary of the first HMO's efforts. Plan dollars would be better spent in that case in seeking inexpensive treatment options rather than in focusing on wellness. However, a cooperative program of wellness, supported throughout the community by all plans, would pay off in the short term for all plans and providers at financial risk. (Longer-term consequences of this and other similar positive strategies are discussed in Chapter 10.)

Plans and providers within a community are often competing for service contracts from the same purchasers. Each purchaser has a different set of information requirements, and each plan or provider has a different way of satisfying the requirements. Thus, X number of purchasers and Y number of plans equals X times Y different formats that must be developed within the community. A cooperative approach to the contracting process could yield a single format followed by all players, with minor variations.

Plans or provider groups may find that their facilities and staff are not readily accessible to a portion of the population they serve. These patients may be in rural areas, inner cities, or institutions, or they may be homebound. Community-wide communications links to serve these patients may aid in their access to information and treatment.

Individual Enterprise Needs

It is difficult to think of anything a single enterprise might need that no other enterprise needs, aside from its own competitive advantage. Healthcare executives may assume that withholding cooperation related to the common goal of information flow will give them that competitive edge. But the edge they gain under those circumstances benefits neither the enterprise, the purchaser, nor the prospective patient. It has nothing to do with providing high-quality care, and it is not sustainable. Enterprises must cooperate at the community level in order to compete effectively.

Individual Physician Needs

Physicians appear to be able to practice their clinical skills quite well in the face of an inefficient, unreliable, untimely, and cumbersome flow of patient information and despite the inaccessibility of essential aspects of medical knowledge. As quality assessment performance measures improve, however, physicians will be held to a higher standard of care. As this begins to happen, they will welcome more accessible patient records and expert advice as indispensable tools for effective clinical practice in both office and hospital.

FROM NEEDS TO INCENTIVES

Although CHINs are complex in design and implementation, the concepts that drive them are quite straightforward, and the solutions bring highly desirable value to the enterprise. The several information needs, collected in the previous section, all point to a universal need at the enterprise level for access to high-quality, reliable information in patient records that may or may not "belong" to the enterprise. For instance, a health plan requires a new member's medical history from his or her former providers. Enterprises also need a more powerful and accessible dynamic medical knowledge base for their physicians and other professional personnel. Further, they need a system of quality assurance that incorporates the quality feedback cycles discussed in Chapter 3, a sensible uniform payment system, and access to potential members for marketing and healthcare. Acknowledging the information-intensive basis of these needs leads inescapably to a solution that includes shared health information networks such as CHINs. More than just networks are needed, however. A collaboratively designed, complex system for information assessment, analysis, and management, including an information distribution network, is called for. In other words, enterprises need CHINs.

Healthcare executives may acknowledge that these system and information needs are legitimate, even though they have no personal motivation to collaborate in meeting these needs. After all, interenterprise systems are expensive and difficult to construct under even the best of circumstances, and the potential for loss of institutional privacy is not a welcome prospect. If motivation internal to the enterprise is guarded, however, external incentives abound, such as the reporting requirements of state and federal government.

The need, then, is for a set of CHIN capabilities that minimizes healthcare executives' concerns while meeting internal and external demands for information. The next section discusses valuable capabilities that can be achieved with currently available technology and enterprise expertise. Most do not involve issues of patient privacy, and none calls for sharing data of competitive value with other community enterprises. Collectively, these incentives could move previously reluctant enterprises to embrace CHINs.

INCENTIVES TO COLLABORATE

The most useful incentives motivating healthcare executives to collaborate in the development of CHINs would come from an inner conviction that their enterprises are an integral part of a larger system that can function only with their full cooperation. That system is being threatened today by its own complexity and weight; its weaknesses are being exploited through fragmentation of its assets. It can be restored to its full functionality only by pooling resources and making the effort to create an infrastructure that will enable all enterprises to work for a successful future.

Meeting System Needs

A healthcare enterprise such as a health plan, provider group, or hospital is almost a microcosm of the healthcare system as a whole. Consider that, like the healthcare system, each enterprise has a need for its own infrastructure within which to manage and carry out its missions. It must have mechanisms for information flow, planning, tracking utilization, professional education, patient care, quality assurance, feedback from departments and staff, and the management of change. The enterprise depends on its individual departments to cooperate in these infrastructural activities. The departments do cooperate because the enterprise executives and department personnel know that the enterprise cannot succeed without that cooperation.

Try to imagine how the enterprise would function if each department conducted its business independently, to the extent that each had its own unconnected management information system and refused to contribute to a common medical record. The enterprise would be unable to coordinate patient care, maintain patient records, or collect treatment information for billing, statistical reports, or quality assurance programs.

This is precisely the state of affairs in the healthcare system as a whole. In a move to cut costs, the patient care and payment subsystems are in the process of divorcing themselves from research and education. Feedback between major segments of the system, such as quality assurance and medical education, is almost nonexistent, as is any form of communication for common purposes such as resource allocation. Health plan and provider enterprises no longer support each other in shared community programs. Instead, they are competing: not constructively to provide the best care or the most access, but by undercutting each other's prices using methods that create extensive system dissonance. What the healthcare system most needs is cooperative contributions to solutions from its individual enterprises.

Even with sound incentives in place, many system needs cannot be met at the community level. A community alone, for instance, cannot create a healthcare system infrastructure, plan and manage system resources, educate professionals, accredit their institutions, or install a common system for financing care. However, communities where healthcare stakeholders have learned to work together toward common community goals have a head start in joining with other, similarly experienced communities to work toward state and national goals.

Enterprise-Oriented Community Incentives

This section expands on ideas introduced as "community-specific needs" to show how these needs can become incentives to enterprises. Community healthcare enterprises surely must contemplate their futures with uncertainty. They can not be sure who their institutional partners will be tomorrow, which doctors will be part of their plans, or which patients they will be serving. Each time a change occurs in any of these arenas, a series of further changes is triggered within the enterprise, ranging from phone book revision to schedule and database modification. Since this can and often does happen to every healthcare enterprise in the community, it makes good sense to find common solutions for the advantage of each enterprise in the community. Ways in which information technology can help minimize the effects of ever-changing affiliations and members is the topic of the next several sections. While each of the identified individual incentives may not be sufficient to justify community collaboration for information flow, collectively even the most basic initiatives become visibly worthwhile.

Reaffiliation

Because institutions and partners within an enterprise need to communicate—and most enterprises believe that this communication should occur via an electronic telecommunications link—each organizational reconfiguration, bar none, requires that the enterprise information infrastructure undergo reconfiguration. This infrastructure is usually an *enterprise network* that links only the enterprise's current affiliates and perhaps its payors. Thus, whenever a new hospital, outpatient facility, laboratory, or pharmacy affiliates, the enterprise's management information systems need to accommodate the change. The need is for constant communication, as often vast amounts of information need to change hands and be jointly maintained. This information ranges from personnel rosters and policies through inventories, formularies, and services to master patient indexes, databases, and even patient records.

Currently, the substantial cost of the new or altered information flow must enter into the business decision to affiliate, but this need not be the burden it is today. If all community enterprises were to routinely share information among their affiliates by participating in a health information network such as a CHIN, then even when the partners changed, information flow would become a background issue: all providers in the community would already be linked to the CHIN.

Previously a CHIN was likened to a telephone system offering communitywide communication. Now consider adding to the communication system an intelligent postal system whereby—simply put—an enterprise specifies the information that needs to be shared and the system finds and delivers it according to pre-agreed rules. Any kind of information could be the subject of such sharing arrangements.

Physician mobility

The professional staff of every healthcare enterprise in the community is drawn from the same pool of physicians—the physicians who live and work in the community. Physicians may be captive to a single enterprise or, more likely, an individual physician, group, or clinic may see patients from many different health plans or payors. Healthcare executives know that physician affiliations are subject to change, so it makes good sense to minimize the work of all enterprises individually by maintaining a community database of physician information available to anyone who needs the information. Such a database would contain items like demographic information, education, licenses and certifications, experience, special strengths, honors, and affiliations.

The database would be a constant community resource, regardless of which enterprises a physician affiliated with. While enterprises need this kind of information about all their physicians, the physicians themselves need this information about their colleagues for purposes such as referrals. Members of plans also could gain access to the information to help them select plans and providers, as could resource planners who need to be certain the community has the number and kind of physicians it needs. Physicians in other communities could have access to the database for referral information as well, and either graduating or established physicians from other communities could find out from the database whether their particular skills are needed in the community.

Mobility of member populations

Although the member population of a health plan may experience considerable turnover from year to year, the population base from which members are drawn still comprises the people who live in the community. That is, all community enterprises draw their members from the same population base. The institutional continuity lost when large changes in membership occur benefits no one in the short run, except perhaps the purchaser who presumably has changed plans to save money. At a minimum, plans have the headache of purging member records and acquiring patient histories from diverse other providers or generating new ones. Treatments may be interrupted as patients move to new plans and doctors, and wellness and preventive care programs may be disrupted.

A common system through which community information can flow during changes in enrollment would have clear advantages. The orderly administrative transfer of member information and authorizations from one enterprise to another whenever necessary would be of great benefit. Enterprises could work with the commonly available community database to update their own databases by removing members no longer active and adding new ones. Perhaps even more useful, such a system could automatically provide enterprise physicians throughout the community with the new member information.

It should be noted that the orderly transfer of clinically relevant information would be of even greater benefit, but this capability is not classified here as an incentive. Transferring the bulk of patients' clinical information electronically is a complex task that is better considered as a goal, rather than an incentive to develop a CHIN.

The benefits of a community database do not stop with the enrollment period. A reasonable subset of population information, such as demographics, allergies, and major diagnoses, commonly available to all enterprises through a health information network such as a CHIN would have great value as a resource planning and marketing tool and as a planning aid to target community wellness programs.

Consumer-Oriented Community Incentives

Many community-directed incentives go beyond lifting the burdens of shifting relationships. These include a variety of community outreach programs of value to all providers and plans that seek to achieve a healthier population as economically as possible. Several examples of such programs are given below. Each of these programs may be difficult for a single health plan to justify, but when they are part of a larger effort to enhance information flow for the entire community, the value they add for the enterprise is high.

Communication for community health

Members' involvement in managing their own health is an important practical matter for health plans. However, when enterprises currently want to reach their members through the mass media with public health messages, educational materials, and wellness programs, they may find that they are in fact providing these services to the entire community at their own expense. With a CHIN, consumers can selectively have computer-based access to patient educational programs, wellness information, advice lines, or even electronic interaction with providers for scheduling appointments or discussing medical problems. Since every enterprise has the same need, community education and consumer access also offer a powerful arena for collaboration.

Telemedicine

Healthcare executives whose enterprises serve rural or institutionalized populations find that the tools of telemedicine have cost-effective potential for improving the care of patients in these settings. Currently, telecommunications costs are quite high and the necessary quality of telecommunications service is not yet generally available. However, communities where telemedicine seems to be a practical approach should start now to begin planning and working toward the legislation or regulation needed to bring about the required telecommunications capability at an affordable price (The Telecommunications and Health Care Advisory Committee 1997).

Shared community programs

Healthcare enterprises have much to gain from closer linkages with many other health-oriented community entities. For example, schools are a great place to reach students with a range of preventive services, wellness programs, and health and medical information resources. But most schools are not in a position to forge such links with a single provider. Instead, they—and community funding agencies— would favor a collaboration of the major community providers to establish the electronic linkages that would facilitate development of shared clinical and information facilities. Even with shared facilities, each plan or provider could have access to records for its member students only.

A rural county in North Carolina plans to develop a system that links county social services information and school records with medical records to coordinate more complete care of children.

Children of all ages will benefit from the resulting information flow that advises teachers of health or social problems, for instance, or advises doctors of school and social problems.

Collaboration in several other arenas, facilitated by the electronic linkages of a health information network, include

- public screening programs for conditions such as elevated blood pressure or cholesterol, or assessment of physical fitness, diet, and other risk factors;

- linkages to home healthcare agencies to facilitate the continuum of care;

- shared environmental or industrial risk databases for the identification of problem areas and affected individuals;

- care for the uninsured as a means of contributing to a healthy community;

- support of telecommunications links into homes to facilitate closer communication with chronically ill patients, to monitor vital signs, and to review medication and other orders; and

- Internet access as a rich health information resource for consumers.

Physician-Oriented Community Incentives

Despite the extensive changes in the organization and financing of healthcare, clinical practice has not changed at the same pace. Physicians naturally might be relieved that this is the case, since so much of their time and resources are consumed just by coping with the administrative and cultural changes imposed by the system. Thus, it is not reasonable to expect that physicians will be motivated to adopt capabilities that will simply add more change without obvious benefits to patient care or office practice. However, clear motivation can be found by helping physicians to cope better with the unavoidable changes that are being externally imposed.

Consider, for instance, that capabilities that would manage a physician's patient database vis-à-vis the plans he or she is affiliated with could go far toward easing administrative headaches. Such a system would automatically advise the doctor's office about each patient's coverage and the specialist to whom that patient may be referred when one is needed. It would also know when preauthorization is required, how to obtain it, and how to bill or account for services rendered according to the guidelines of each plan. Physicians would welcome a readily usable system that saved such large chunks of staff time from record keeping, phone calls, faxing, filing, and looking up information.

Another externally imposed factor that would motivate physicians is the growing emphasis on quality. Management services organizations (MSOs), which may be hired to run group practices or clinics, also frequently negotiate managed care, or capitated care, contracts for their physicians. MSOs increasingly must accept contracts that include a new level of accountability, requiring the doctor to prove the quality of the care he or she delivers. The contracts may even require the physicians to follow specific clinical guidelines aimed at high-quality care.

Once the bar has been raised for standards of care, physicians will surely welcome the technology and tools of a CHIN that make compliance possible. They will need the results of ongoing quality assessment for their practices and for the institutions such as hospitals and plans with which they are affiliated; access to constantly updated guidelines and alerts, preferably integrated into the patient's record so that they can be reviewed as the chart is updated; and better access to the dynamic MKB and continuing education materials such as simulations and tutorials.

Consider the value of physician-hospital linkages as a further example of physician-oriented incentives. If an electronic link exists between hospitals and their affiliated physicians, whether in an integrated delivery system or in a looser arrangement, at a minimum physicians can admit patients, order procedures, review reports or results of tests, and review and sign discharge summaries.

Finally, an electronic link between physicians in the same or different groups would allow electronic consultations by e-mail. It is even possible today for physicians to consult together or attend rounds using videoconferencing facilities built into their office computers and looking at the patient record at the same time.

Payor Incentives

Payors need information related to cost and quality of care. They need utilization and outcomes information not only for their own use, but also for purchasers, such as employers and pension plans, that want to know their healthcare dollars are being well spent. To obtain this information, payors could establish a system within a CHIN for hospitals and doctors that would carry out the common steps of claims processing and reporting utilization and outcomes at that level in the case of health plans. The same CHIN facilities could be used to supply electronically accessible information to providers about patient enrollment, authorizations, and so on.

Information systems are in place in industries throughout the world to account for, manage, and control the processes of financing and payment. It appears to many that the only real barrier to achieving such a fully integrated electronic tracking and payment system in healthcare may be lack of leadership and willingness to collaborate. Health plans active in a community could act even in the absence of national standardization and coordination to ease the burden on providers in their own communities. Since such a system may actually be cost justifiable for payors, some communities may be fortunate to have payors who are willing to install a CHIN specifically for these purposes. Community representatives may even be permitted to have control of the CHIN without having to take the financial risk.

Government-Supplied Incentives

We have seen how recent changes in the healthcare system have created extensive dissonance. These changes range from reallocating system dollars, to radically altering the business incentives in the system, to separating clinical research and professional education from patient care, to exposing physician passivity and apparent powerlessness. From the point of view of citizens, many of these changes cannot be seen in a positive light, and thus they invite government interest and action on behalf of the population.

Precedents for government action to control the healthcare system are abundant. Many states, such as Oregon, have acted to create entirely different systems of care within their boundaries, and other governments, including the federal government, are watching their progress with interest. Almost every state has passed, or at least has introduced legislation to curb health plans' freedom to act. The federal government itself even opened the door to legislating clinical care practices when it dictated standards for practices such as minimum length of stay allowed for new mothers and their babies.

It should be abundantly clear to healthcare executives that government involvement in health services delivery will expand as long as the system continues to move in directions that do not serve the healthcare goals of society. The system has not had a positive impact on access, judging by the number of uninsured Americans. Nor have the changes lowered overall system costs as expected. Prospects are highly likely for such measures as capping profits, setting fees, establishing quality standards, and moving the system more toward a public health orientation.

Whatever form government regulation or legislation takes, we can be sure that it will include ways to monitor compliance. Already groups within the federal government are working toward a National Information Infrastructure (NII) that will include an information infrastructure for healthcare (Fitzmaurice 1994). Such an infrastructure would not only provide the mechanism for the federal government to obtain feedback on the effectiveness of, and compliance with, its programs. At a minimum it would also provide the means for offering universal professional access to research findings and other medical information in the dynamic MKB, as well as offering access to a host of other quality assurance materials such as clinical guidelines and education programs. Further justification for the NII lies in the realm of

- providing a conduit for new types of clinical research such as models that make extensive use of basic data in the CPR, as discussed in Chapter 3;
- offering consumer informatics (health and medical information for consumers) and research; and
- sharing planning resources among providers and policymakers.

How is this an incentive for CHIN development? It is probable that the way individual enterprises, institutions, and providers will connect to the NII will be through CHINs. Those communities whose CHINs are sufficiently mature will likely maintain control of the nature and content of those linkages. In other words, if communities do not begin to implement health information networks, then government will no doubt dictate that it be done "their way."

BEYOND THE BASICS OF COOPERATION

Although the incentives to collaborate in developing health information networks may seem wide ranging and uncoordinated, nothing could be farther from the truth. Every one of them is directed toward health system goals, and when one enterprise works toward these capabilities, it does not affect other community enterprises negatively; instead, all enterprises benefit. These are powerful incentives indeed.

A closer look shows that virtually all of these capabilities are enabled by the same health information networks, or CHINs. Whether the information is for or about physicians, patients, health plan members in general, or community institutions, the same network links the same stakeholders for multiple purposes. Often, the same information, such as patient information, is used to meet multiple needs. It merely needs to be abstracted, analyzed, and presented in different ways. Clearly, the more capabilities that are implemented on a CHIN, and the more it is used, the more the CHIN pays off for the participating enterprises. Also clearly, the CHIN benefits enterprises and the community most fully when *every* major stakeholder is involved and contributing. Only with full participation can the information base for the CHIN be complete and all CHIN benefits be realized.

By cooperating to achieve a systemwide infrastructure, the primary role of health plan and provider enterprises is that of beneficiary. A well-ordered healthcare system can benefit enterprises only when it provides all of the resources and functions they need to deliver the best patient care.

References

Fitzmaurice, J. M. 1994. "Health Care and the NII." Rockville, MD: U.S. Department of Health and Human Services Agency for Health Care Policy and Research.

The Telecommunications and Health Care Advisory Committee. 1997. "Findings and Recommendations." Washington, DC: Federal Telecommunications Commission.

CHAPTER 5

ASSESSING THE VALUE
OF CHIN CAPABILITIES

When CHIN initiators consider the incentives that might lead them to develop a CHIN, they face several dilemmas. They know that the larger the number of stakeholders involved in and relying on the CHIN, the more likely it is to be accepted and succeed. Thus they want to associate themselves with powerful incentives that will attract stakeholders. On the other hand, they do not want to invest time, effort, and money into a CHIN that supports activities characteristic of only a passing healthcare fad.

THE SEARCH FOR
RELEVANCE AND VALUE

Among all of the changes to organization, payment, and care delivery in healthcare, it is hard to tell just which approaches will become, at best, just one of several styles of delivering care, and which changes are an enduring contribution to the delivery of care. The substantial commitment required of participants by even a limited CHIN project means it is highly important to make some kind of assessment of this very issue. For example, many health systems experts believe that, while managed care concepts have a lot to offer healthcare, today's managed care organizations (MCOs) cannot survive in their present mode of giving precedence to money management rather than care enhancement. From a systems perspective, there are sound reasons for this conclusion.

Managed care was originally conceived to improve efficiency in healthcare and raise the level of health of the population. The reasoning was, if a healthcare organization had a limited amount of money to spend, it would reduce organizational waste in all of its forms, including eliminating unnecessary or useless treatments and keeping its patients healthier. In common with virtually all healthcare organizations over the past several years, MCOs, too, have managed to reduce their costs. But designers of managed care concepts never imagined that MCOs would cut costs at the expense of the even more significant goal of ready access to high-quality care. Nor did they imagine that a substantial proportion of the savings would be taken out of the healthcare system in the form of profits for shareholders.

Many MCO practices have already led to challenges by new provider-sponsored groups, by consumers in arbitration and in the courts, and in legislatures. For managed care to succeed, MCOs would need to shift the focus of their guiding value system. They would need to reward clinical quality and become contributing members to the health of the community and the healthcare system as a whole. That is, for all of the reasons cited earlier, they would need to work cooperatively toward community wellness and standards of quality of care, and they would need to participate in the clinical research and teaching aspects of healthcare as well as in patient care.

When establishing CHINs, therefore, it makes sense for communities to base their plans primarily on the underlying needs and goals of the healthcare system. They should avoid setting up CHINs that are dependent for adherents on a particular approach to care delivery. Instead, CHIN features should be of lasting value to the health of the community whether its providers are independent or are affiliated with such enterprises as MCOs or integrated delivery systems.

LONG-TERM VALUE VS. SHORT-TERM MOTIVATION

Because so many healthcare enterprises are trying just to survive under the competitive models prevalent today, it seems that the short term is the only viable focus. Their first questions concern the potential for tangible return on their investment and, understandably, they do not think they can get involved in potentially expensive diversions from the business of survival. Their problems are not at all incompatible with participation in a CHIN, however, as many possible CHIN activities can yield benefits. These benefits in the short term would be in the form of new cost avoidance.

Changes in healthcare are putting pressure on enterprises to do things that were never necessary in the traditional healthcare system. Now these enterprise changes must not only be made to compete and to lower costs, but also to carry out the patient care mission. Each of these new kinds of activities involves putting in place new mechanisms with their attendant costs. Consider the following examples, all of which are information intensive:

- To compete, enterprises must provide extensive information to potential or current purchasers about services, costs, and quality. To reach potential new members such as seniors, they must employ market techniques like TV, print media, and direct mail advertising, and even call on prospective members personally.

- To lower costs, enterprises must provide more extensive educational opportunities for members, reengineer business processes, and track their physicians' activities very closely.

- In terms of patient care, since hospitalized patients are not staying as long, the need exists for more extensive follow-up and coordination of home care and outpatient care.

- The information burden imposed by the accreditation process is more onerous than ever.

- Managed care, whether capitated or not, places a heavy new burden on physicians and other outpatient providers such as home care agencies. These groups must keep track of the details of a number of plans and correctly match patients to plans, and they are accountable to the plans for both the care and the cost of the care they deliver.

These kinds of activities are the duty of individual enterprises, but it is important to note that every healthcare enterprise in the community faces the same challenges and costs. To achieve cost avoidance, time and money can be saved when many of these new information-intensive activities are developed cooperatively by several enterprises in the community using a CHIN. At the same time, because the activities would be CHIN-based and collaboratively developed, they would serve as building blocks for the global vision of the CHIN: to raise the level of health and improve the level of care in the long term.

ASKING THE RIGHT QUESTIONS

In the conceptualization/planning stage, as noted earlier, prospective CHIN initiators rightly want to know

- Who is the CHIN customer?
- What is the business case?
- What is the information content being transmitted (Williams 1996)?

Now these questions can be seen for what they really are. They are surrogates for questions about the value of the activities that community CHIN participants are contemplating. The twin dilemma of wanting to appeal to potential participants for shared development costs, while maintaining relevance in the healthcare system for the long term, directly addresses the need for connection between the healthcare goals and problems of the evolving system discussed in Chapter 2, and the motivating and provocative incentives discussed in Chapter 4. This chapter shows how potential CHIN collaborators can determine just how viable their candidate CHIN activities will be in the long run.

THE TRADITIONAL VIEW

Guidance for the critical strategic planning issue of long-term CHIN viability is hard to find in the CHIN literature. Experts apparently believed that potential partners wanted to do everything one could do with a CHIN. Healthcare executives were assumed to be willing to work toward the ultimate full connectivity allowed by technology, and selection of the initial capabilities to be developed was generally considered to be entirely a practical matter rather than one of the highest strategic importance. Thus, a decision on direction was likely to be made based on such factors as who would contribute the most resources, who would own and manage the CHIN, and what technology and expertise were available.

Wakerly defines strategic goals in terms of benefits back to the participating enterprises (Wakerly 1994). These goals are given as capabilities and transactions within these three functionalities, roughly in increasing order of technical complexity:

1. Administrative/financial (claims processing, orders, results)
2. Clinical (data storage, access, and analysis)
3. Operational (appointment scheduling, remote patient monitoring, imaging).

He also offers extensive practical advice on such topics as styles of CHIN ownership, vendor selection, technology architectures, available enterprise application expertise, the need for project management resource expertise, and implementation guidelines.

The COMNET Society report describes CHINs in terms of their ownership, management, funding source, operational entity, and functionality. Functionality is described as occurring in one of these five areas:

1. Administrative (messaging, demographics, ID cards);
2. Clinical (orders, results, referrals, CPR, telemedicine);

3. Financial (eligibility, referral authorization, claims processing);
4. Central data repository (population-based analyses); and
5. Educational (teleconferencing, information services) (Community Medical Network Society 1995).

The report further proposes the interesting idea that all information technology use in enterprises is part of their evolutionary path of development toward a CHIN. In other words, each is a CHIN-in-progress. The Society recognized the importance of benefit and buy-in for all participants, but again the focus is on return and benefit to the partners.

Both of these useful references reinforce the general assumption that the ultimate goal and result of CHIN developments today will be the mature CHIN, which embodies full-blown integration of information technology into healthcare. This goal is endorsed, even though initially planned functionality may have little to do with that goal. It is because of this goal assumption that many CHINs skipped the strategic planning phase entirely and moved directly to the exciting activities of recruiting partners, raising money, and delving into the wonders of available technology options.

TOOLS FOR A VALUE-BASED ASSESSMENT

CHIN charters tend to be broadly visionary, often espousing healthcare system goals. The challenge comes with defining the specific initial steps tht are perceived as valuable to potential participants and that also serve as building blocks, or at least stepping stones, to the more global CHIN vision.

Actual or potential CHINs need to take the essential step of assessing the long-term viability and value of their plans. They need to be certain that they have found the optimal set of initial functionality that will yield the essential short-term benefits while ensuring that long-term value is also served. Two key mindsets are essential to the process.

First, healthcare enterprises of all kinds must understand that an information system cannot in the short run be justified as a profit center, although some costs should be recouped in the long run through selling information and offering value-added services. Information systems will increasingly continue to be an indispensable part of the cost of doing business, however. With appropriate planning and management information systems investments can meet realistic expectations (Glaser 1997).

Second, the goals of healthcare, and therefore the goals of any enterprise in healthcare, including CHINs, are generally taken to be the provision of good health and high-quality, affordable medical care for all. Further, CHIN capabilities that serve these health system goals serve all stakeholders equally, whereas capabilities that serve enterprise-specific goals do not.

This section shows ways in which CHIN planners can use a simple two-way table to begin an assessment of the feasibility of contemplated CHIN functions in terms of their long-term viability and value to the community. Three simple tools are needed:

1. a wish list of the candidate capabilities, functionalities, or applications being considered for the CHIN;

2. the healthcare system mission statement (the basis of a mature CHIN), expressed as discrete goals; and

3. a two-way table where a reasonable value assessment of each capability can be recorded and weighed.

We begin by analyzing the diverse incentives described in Chapter 4 after first translating them into CHIN capabilities. The analysis results in a value assessment table that shows the relevance of the selected CHIN capabilities to healthcare goals. Keep in mind that a distinctive feature of this list is that all the capabilities are readily doable with currently available technology and typical enterprise expertise, and that most do not involve issues of patient privacy. None calls for sharing data of competitive value with other community enterprises.

Since the incentives were categorized by the stakeholders they would benefit, the list of capabilities based on the incentives is broader than most CHINs would use. Typical CHIN planning initially considers only those capabilities that have short-term benefit for one or more of the partner enterprises. Table 5.1 shows the value assessment table with capabilities listed in approximately the same categories as were used in Chapter 4 for easy reference. The column headings are health system goals:

- to improve population health;
- to maintain/improve quality of care;
- to assure individual access to care, communication, and information; and
- to simplify administration or reduce/avoid costs (possibly through reengineering in addition to simple replacement of manual functions).

Not surprisingly, most of the capabilities that were identified as incentives for physician participation would have the effect of improving quality of medical care. Also to be expected, the incentives

Table 5.1   Value Assessment Table

Capabilities	Health	Quality	Access	Administration/ Finance
Values				
Community Oriented				
Plan information database			X	X
Doctor information database		X		X
Population information database	X	X	X	X
Provider information database				X
Information regarding community resources	X		X	X
Patient access to medical knowledge base	X	X	X	
Internet access for patients	X	X	X	
Medline access for patients		X	X	
Public health messages for patients	X		X	
"Disease-related" programs for community		X	X	
Indigent care			X	
Rural telemedicine			X	
Urban telemedicine			X	
Wellness programs for community	X			
Connection with schools	X			
Connection with community agencies	X			
Physician/Provider Oriented				
E-mail: doctors—patients		X	X	
E-mail: doctors—doctors		X		
Videoconferencing: doctors—doctors		X		
Results reporting		X		X
Inpatient orders				X
Admitting/appointments				X
Discharge summaries				X
Plan guidelines for doctors		X		
Doctors access medical knowledge base		X		
Internet access for staff		X		
Medline access for staff		X		
Public health messages for staff		X		
Community development guidelines		X		
Connection with homes		X		
Financing Oriented				
Common report for purchasers				X
Claims processing				X
Plan information for provider				X
Doctors report to plans				X
Feedback regarding quality to purchasers		X		

to payors and purchasers would lead to improvements and efficiencies in financing and paying for healthcare.

The most compelling cluster, however, is in the community-oriented capabilities. These are capabilities that would benefit the community population and healthcare enterprises in general. Collectively, these capabilities are aligned with all of the health system values; most strongly, they improve access to care, and most of them also support improvement in the community's baseline health, the quality of patient care, efficiency in the system, or all three. Most of the impact of access at these early stages is in access to information and communication channels rather than in access to care. The exception is the area of telemedicine, where actual care not previously available may be provided.

AN EXAMPLE OF A CHIN VALUE ASSESSMENT

The Wisconsin Health Information Network is generally considered to be the first successful CHIN in the United States. Founded in 1992, the statewide WHIN is an outgrowth of a successful enterprise network. The functionality selected for WHIN early in its strategic planning is the basis for Table 5.2, where WHIN's planned functionality is assessed against healthcare system values.

WHIN's planned functionality primarily affects the administration and financing aspects of the system, which is surely where the clearest short-term business case for a CHIN can be made. The agenda also makes a start on some measures to improve quality of care through improved availability of information. Most important for the future, however, is the extensive connectivity that WHIN can achieve through the state. As will be shown in Chapter 6, connectivity is an important building block toward a mature CHIN.

WEIGHTED VALUE ASSESSMENT

Although Tables 5.1 and 5.2 indicate merely the substantial presence or absence of a value, it is also possible to assign *weights* that assess the *degree of relevancy* of capabilities to healthcare values. Table 5.3 shows a portion of the information in Table 5.1, where a scale of 1 to 3 (from lowest to highest relevance) indicates the relative value of a capability with respect to each system value.

From Table 5.3 CHIN planners can conclude that community databases of many types tend to have considerable administrative value, while information gotten to consumers can positively affect the other three goals of improving health, access, and quality of care. In general, when information flow to consumers is unidirectional,

Table 5.2   WHIN Functionality Value Assessment Table

	Values			
Functionality	**Health**	**Quality**	**Access**	**Administration/ Finance**
Patient Inquiries				
Patient census				X
Patient demographics				X
Patient searches				X
Medical records abstracts				X
Medications ordered		X		
Inpatient/outpatient search		X		X
Utilization review		X		
Patient eligibility				X
Process Claims				
Submit claims				X
Check status				X
Notify resolution				X
Eligibility				X
Report Results				
Transcribed reports				X
Laboratory results				X
Radiology results				X
Radiology images		X		
Send Information				
Messages				X
Bulletin board				X
Out-fax				X
Referrals		X		X
Advice regarding insurance enrollment				X
Claims processing information				X
Medical information and library aervices		X		
Future				
Prescription transmission		X		
Attestation				X

Table 5.3 Weighted Value Assessment Table

Capabilities	Health	Quality	Access	Administration/Finance
Community Oriented				
Plan information database			1	2
Doctor information database		1		3
Population information database	1	1	1	3
Provider information database				2
Information regarding community resources	2		1	1
Patient access to medical knowledge base	2	1	1	
Internet access for patients	2	1	1	
Medline access for patients		1	1	
Public health messages for patients	1		1	
"Disease-related" programs for community		1	1	
E-mail: doctors—patients		2	2	
Indigent care			3	
Rural telemedicine			3	

such as when they use Medline, impact is minimal. When two-way communication is established between patients and caregivers, however, messages are reinforced, feedback is available, and impact is greater. And impact on the serious problems of quality and access is greatest when actual patient care is altered.

Note that these weights are not the same as priorities, although they should certainly be key elements in setting priorities. Setting priorities is a complex determination involving acuity of need, cost, resources, feasibility, and a host of other factors. For example, telemedicine is a high-profile capability that can positively affect the access problems of some geographic regions. But the essential high-speed communications technology is prohibitively expensive today, especially in rural areas. Moreover, telemedicine is an organizationally complex and labor-intensive process. Thus, assigning it a high priority will be a complex decision involving many factors.

The capabilities and values used in Tables 5.1 and 5.3 are generic. In particular, the values chosen as desirable are attributable to the healthcare system as a whole, but a CHIN's goals may be a subset of these or entirely different. They may be phrased, for instance, in terms of educational achievement if the CHIN is being established primarily for educational purposes.

It is a good idea in some circumstances to cast the potential CHIN capabilities against at least two sets of values, generating two or more tables. The first table should use the values of the healthcare system to ground the CHIN in the big picture of healthcare. The other table(s) can use community goals or the stated CHIN goals as its values. This step prepares CHIN planners for the next phase of analysis, which uses techniques based on building blocks to show whether, and how, planned CHIN capabilities are actually linked to goals.

References · · · · · · · · · · · ·

Community Medical Network (COMNET) Society. 1995. *COMNET's HIN Market Directory, 1996 edition.* Atlanta, GA: Community Medical Network Society.

Glaser, J. P. 1997. "Beware 'Return on Investment.'" *Healthcare Informatics* 14 (6): 134–8.

Wakerly, R. T. (ed.). 1994. *Community Health Information Networks.* Chicago: American Hospital Publishing.

Williams, S. 1996. "Florida: Systems Integrator is Key to Success." *Infocare* (September/October) 54–56.

CHAPTER 6

CHIN BUILDING BLOCKS

The process shown in the previous chapter assesses the relevance of planned CHIN capabilities to health system, community, and CHIN goals. That process may be most helpful for an individual CHIN as a way to highlight potential dissonances where further analysis and planning are needed. The next discussion, on *CHIN building blocks*, shows how such dissonances can be further examined and resolved.

CHIN building blocks are the key components of a CHIN that contribute to, and are essential to, the whole. Ideally, each planned or actual CHIN capability is a building block that becomes an integral and essential part of the CHIN. Since most CHINs begin with a focus on administrative and financial efficiencies, the discussion of building blocks begins there also.

CAPABILITIES THAT SUPPORT GOALS

Basing a new CHIN on administrative and financing efficiencies is certainly acceptable when these are understood to be the goal of the CHIN. After all, this is where a tangible return on investment is most likely to be demonstrated—a very important factor for some CHIN investors. However, problems occur when the goals of the CHIN are stated to be improvement of the health of the population and the quality of medical care in the community, but the capabilities chosen for implementation cannot be shown to lead to these goals. In this case, the CHIN too often simply adds to the dissonance in the system. It adds dissonance because, as a system itself, the CHIN lacks one of the key aspects of successful systems—*congruence of goals* for all elements of the system. In this case, failure of congruence occurs when some partners expect the CHIN to fulfill a set of spoken or written goals having to do with quality, while others are working toward unspoken goals or hidden agendas having to do with administrative efficiency.

THE BUILDING BLOCK ANALYSIS

Clearly, it is in the best interests of a CHIN that wants to achieve longevity, as well as in the best interests of every one of its actual or potential partners and stakeholders, to achieve congruence of goals. But far too many CHIN planners, in their zeal to get started, have succumbed to the lure of overselling the impact of planned capabilities. That is, the promised goals clearly would not result from these particular planned capabilities. Big dreams are a must, because a mature CHIN can help fulfill big dreams for healthcare, but getting off to a well-reasoned start is also a must.

Building block analysis is a technique for identifying sets of goals and starting points that are compatible and realistic. It works in two ways. First, a *bottom-up analysis* for CHINs with firm plans begins with proposed capabilities and goals and looks for assurance of a match. Second, a *top-down analysis* begins with goals and then works down to define that set of capabilities required to achieve the goals. The initial CHIN capabilities should then devolve from that set.

These are very simple techniques that may seem obvious, something that everyone does automatically whenever he or she is confronted with expensive and powerful decisions. However simple the bottom-up/top-down analysis may be, it is difficult to find CHINs that show evidence of having consciously gone through this process. It would also be difficult to find a group of CHIN investors that would not benefit from such an analysis. Thus, it is worth taking the time to explore the building block process here.

Bottom-Up Building Block Analysis

CHIN mission statements often tend to equate the achievement of administrative efficiencies early in the CHIN project with improved quality of healthcare in the later stages of CHIN development. After all, quality is so important that, not surprisingly, almost every CHIN wants to have improved quality of care as a goal. There is little logical flow of thought, however, to show that commonly planned administrative initiatives have any direct or even indirect bearing on improvements in quality of care. That is, the currently planned capabilities do not seem to be building blocks toward the goals of the CHIN.

The following are two examples of a simple bottom-up building block analysis of a CHIN's plans. The focus of both examples is on discriminating between activities leading to the goal of administrative efficiencies and those leading to the goal of improved quality of care. The techniques, which could be applied to any set of capabilities and goals, consist of (1) identifying the fact that evidence is needed to show that certain capabilities will in fact eventually yield the promised results and (2) finding and evaluating such evidence, which could take many forms ranging from pilot projects or studies in the literature, to calculations, consensus—or common sense.

Administrative efficiencies without quality improvement

A CHIN may propose to improve quality through administrative efficiencies by providing an electronic link between hospitals and doctors for such purposes as admitting patients, ordering tests, reporting test results, or delivering discharge summaries for review and "signature." The underlying assumption is that, if doctors could spend less time creating, finding, and reviewing such documents, they would spend more time with their patients, thereby improving quality of care. Or they would spend more time keeping up with their professional reading, which also would lead to improved care. In fact, however, if the amount of time saved is significant, doctors will more likely see more patients, rather than change their practice styles. Furthermore, although it is intuitively attractive to assume that more reading or more time spent with each patient will translate into a higher quality of care, these off-hand techniques would more likely prove to be exercises in wishful thinking. A carefully crafted program of feedback to the physician about his or her work, accompanied by targeted educational measures to change behavior, is more likely to improve quality of care.

The foregoing example does offer at least one relationship to future quality-directed functionality: the telecommunications link between hospitals and doctors, established for administrative purposes, can be used for quality improvement as well. However, if the CHIN is doing nothing to identify and develop the other building blocks of quality improvement, then the value of that connectivity for quality improvement is negated. The second example illustrates this point.

Administrative efficiencies with quality improvement

Consider another CHIN, such as California's Healthcare Data Information Corp., where administrative efficiencies are the first planned capabilities, with quality improvement as a longer-term goal (Bazzoli 1996). The quality improvement goal in this case, although unspecified, might be to implement the quality assurance cycles introduced in Chapter 3 into the community. Recall that the essential element of those cycles is a symbiotic information relationship between healthcare enterprises and the dynamic MKB. That is, the physicians associated with the enterprises have an ongoing need for information from the knowledge base, and the knowledge base in turn needs feedback and fresh information from the enterprises to support research, planning, and further development of guidelines and educational materials.

Clearly the quality goal is too complex to be immediately achievable, but some CHIN resources need to be devoted to developing its special building blocks, as evidence that the CHIN really considers it a valid goal. The readily achievable quality building blocks, which are useful and relatively economical capabilities in their own right, are electronic access for physicians to the MKB, educational programs, and collegial communication (e-mail). The electronic access for physicians is an example of a capability useful in both administrative efficiency and quality improvement.

Examples of the essential quality assurance building blocks that need more time for development are a Central Data Repository (CDR) that would contain clinical records for research or for a system of community guideline development. Implementing a CDR raises many of the same issues as a computer-based patient record, such as the need for both medical terminology and technological standards and new information security measures. Issues like these, as well as community guideline development, require extensive and close collaboration among CHIN partners. While one cannot expect a tangible return on investment from such building blocks, they are an essential part of the cost of doing business through a CHIN and of moving toward a mature CHIN.

Healthcare executives who are contemplating affiliation with a CHIN need to make analyses like these to at least this depth and to be alert to the potential for later dissonance when obvious steps are missing from the CHIN plan. Even though the steps between the initial capabilities and realization of goals may be many and complex, CHIN planners should have a good idea of what these steps are, how and when they can and will be accomplished, and how to communicate this information effectively to CHIN partners. If healthcare executives are not satisfied with the logic, they should consider this a signal to seek changes. Once any problems have been identified, goals can be clarified and capabilities can be changed to match and lead to goals.

Top-Down Building Block Analysis

In this case community CHIN planners begin the analysis with healthcare goals that they believe can be facilitated using information technology that links enterprises and other stakeholders in the community. All of the examples that follow are hypothetical. Each example shows how capabilities must be designed to match community goals. They also show that goals probably will not be met if capabilities are chosen on some other basis.

A community wellness program

The major community hospitals in a medium-sized midwestern city have been working together for years in a purchasing cooperative and in maintaining a common computer-based roster of physicians. Key staff at several of the hospitals became alarmed last year at the apparently increasing number of preventable medical problems they were treating. They decided to work together on a community-wide education campaign that they hoped would reverse that trend. After studies to determine which health problems to tackle first, they identified three major categories of tasks:

- developing a marketing strategy to sell "wellness" to the community;

- finding or creating, and then delivering, the educational materials; and

- obtaining feedback to track progress and modify their program for further impact.

Such an information-intensive program of activity naturally led them to consider using a health information network, and they selected the CHIN concept, since their project was for the use and benefit of the entire community. Research showed that entertainment, repetition, and reward are key factors in changing behavior, so these became the focus of the first task of developing their marketing strategy.

For the second task, the largest available body of information for consumers was determined to be accessible on the World Wide Web over the Internet. Since the project would have to provide almost universal connectivity to make the consumer-oriented information available, planners decided to leverage that connectivity by using Internet technology as the primary means of delivering the remaining educational programs they would have to create. In addition to computers in homes, computers for accessing the materials on the Internet were planned for public places such as libraries, schools, churches, health clubs, and even mobile vans.

Obtaining feedback to track progress in an entire community was accomplished primarily through the CHIN. When educational programs were used, this information was recorded in a voluntary communitywide population database. Impact of the programs was measured two ways. First, the same terminals used to present educational materials were used also for pretest and periodic follow-up questionnaires about health status. Second, the same hospital patient databases and processes that led to discovery of the problem in the first place were analyzed on a continuing basis for evidence that the desired behavioral changes had occurred.

Of course, they enlisted schools, libraries, community centers, and newspapers as non-Internet delivery and evaluation mechanisms, too. They even created a great community comic book hero called Megakid, who was the hero of the videogame rewards dispensed on successful completion of educational modules and questionnaires. The support of the entire community, including businesses and government agencies, was critical to the success of the project.

The building blocks designed or acquired for this project included

- public and public institutions' connectivity to Internet resources;
- establishment of a population health database;
- curriculum with imported and original educational materials;
- a project management center (housed at one of the hospitals); and
- extensive community support and cooperation.

These building blocks can be leveraged again and again by using them to deliver additional health-related programs. The connectivity can also be used for other purposes, such as school health records or even non–health related academic access to the Internet. Although for this project, participation in the population database is voluntary, the database could be expanded to become an important planning tool for both healthcare enterprises and other community agencies.

Improved community health was the goal of this CHIN, but if early capabilities implemented with the CHIN had been primarily to connect hospitals with doctors' offices, this project could not have happened. The reason is that the connectivity building blocks needed for this project were for public access, rather than for professional access. As a result of this investment, however, the community also has a formidable process that includes curriculum, educational, and testing materials, which are probably marketable to other communities. Finally, the impetus for the project came from the goal, and multiple stakeholders in the community were active in using a CHIN to create value.

A community quality program

Several health plans share in the use of the only three regional hospitals serving the eastern half of a thinly populated western state. It is a beautiful state that attracts strong, healthy, independent people— and also highly independent doctors. By the time a doctor and patient decide a hospital stay is warranted, the patient is often much sicker than he or she ought to be. Injuries and chronic diseases are a particular problem. Frustrated by the unnecessary suffering and costs, the health plans decided to collaborate on an aggressive program to change the admitting practices of the physicians. Armed with aggregate hospital statistics that showed the egregiousness of the problem, and further armed with a jointly developed office authorization and payment system as an incentive, they persuaded a substantial majority of the widely scattered doctors to participate in a quality improvement program aimed at earlier hospital admission. The tools needed were these:

- a project management office (at one of the plan headquarters);
- telecommunications connectivity between the physicians' offices, hospitals, and the project management office;
- a set of guidelines regarding hospital admission, including transportation, that were specifically designed to meet the needs of the geographic area;
- simulations (case-based training materials) that involved caring for patients like the ones they see most often;
- e-mail communication for community physicians with hospital staff specialists representing each of the plans;
- Internet access to electronically available professional resources such as on-line journals and Medline; and
- a custom office payment system.

Reliable telecommunications connectivity was expensive to achieve, but the cost was leveraged by using it for both the authorization and payment system, which the plans wanted the doctors to use anyway, and the quality admissions project. To measure the success of the program, project managers have been monitoring the extent of physicians' use and their evaluation of the various tools. Analyses of the same hospital databases that brought the problems to light in the first place should show a pattern of earlier admissions that are leading to better patient outcomes and a lower cost of treatment. Future plans call for the physicians' access to their hospitalized patients' records— when the hospitals automate them.

The building blocks needed and used for this project were the connectivity among the hospitals and rural physicians, the custom

office payment system, the guideline development process, the guidelines and simulations, and Internet access.

A community access program

Three huge teaching hospitals—a public, a private nonprofit, and a
for profit—dominate the landscape of a crowded inner city. Despite
the plethora of medical resources in residents' back yards, access to
healthcare was becoming an explosive civic issue. A substantial part
of the community was indigent. Furthermore, even citizens with
healthcare coverage were overusing the emergency rooms because
of the shortage of primary care locations. The hospitals decided to
work cooperatively on changing the access patterns for the covered
population and, with the organizational and financial support of the
city, on creating access for the indigent population.

More primary care locations were essential so, after much study
and analysis, the project decided to establish 24-hour storefront
clinics every three blocks in the residential areas. These were staffed
primarily by interns and residents eager for primary care experience. Transportation was provided from the neighborhood clinics to
specialty clinics and back as necessary. Record keeping for so many
small locations would have been a logistics nightmare, except that the
hospitals were already working to implement a CHIN and a common
master patient index (MPI) to link their far-flung patient databases.
The new clinics were simply added to the CHIN, so this project
became a realistic pilot project for the CHIN and the MPI design.
The clinics would treat anyone who walked in, including the records-
averse. As a condition of its financial participation, however, the city
required that treatment records for the population with no insurance
be maintained and accessible.

The building blocks were the connectivity of the clinics with the
CHIN in development; a simple version of one of the medical centers'
accounting systems, which would handle the financial record keeping
and billing for the clinics; and, most important, the new and badly
needed clinics. The work on this project could be leveraged to develop
a more complete population database for planning and health services
research, one of the hallmarks of a mature CHIN.

In each of these cases, the CHIN capabilities are rather simple,
but they have high impact for the community in terms of addressing
its most pressing healthcare problems. Also in the latter two cases,
capabilities in administration and financing were an integral part of
the quality and access project. As noted before, a CHIN becomes
most valuable when it is used for multiple purposes. The advantages
of starting with simple CHIN capabilities of demonstrable impact

on community health goals is that many of the issues surrounding more complex uses of CHINs are avoided. Some of these issues, such as system security, patient privacy, or the need for a computer-based medical record, are discussed in the next chapter.

CAPABILITY, BUILDING BLOCK, OR GOAL?

It is important not to get too bogged down in terminology, because the real difference among a capability, a building block, and a goal is relative and may even be substantially a question of timing. As a simple rule of thumb, capabilities seem to be simple and short term, while building blocks also include things that take a little longer and may incorporate one or several capabilities without being an end in themselves. CHIN goals, then, would be major accomplishments that contribute substantially to the health of the community.

In one analysis, a given functionality may be considered a capability, while in another, it may be considered a building block or even a goal. Consider as an example the CPR. Some portions of patient records such as diagnoses, procedures, and test results have been automated for years, and sending this information over a CHIN is a popular capability. Those who do so in fact often claim to be transporting medical records. On the other hand, medical informaticians consider the development of a CPR to be an unrealized goal, because so many have spent a professional lifetime trying to achieve a complete CPR. For a mature CHIN, however, the CPR is not a goal, but a vital tool and building block used to facilitate good medical care and contribute to the MKB.

THE NEXT STEPS

Just as the sections above examined the proposed building blocks of CHINs, so these processes themselves are building blocks in the CHIN planning process. The *assessment of relative value* of planned capabilities to the goals of the CHIN or community, the healthcare system, or both is the first step. The *bottom-up building block analysis* then provides a way to decide whether and how a cluster of planned capabilities actually can or will lead to stated goals. Finally, for CHINs that want to actually begin with goals and then select the capabilities needed to achieve them, the *top-down building block analysis* is used.

Besides these specific analyses, there are a number of overarching principles that should also be incorporated into capability planning. Common sense says that it will be necessary to exercise scope control by selecting a probably small subset of all possible and desirable capabilities or applications. When resources are limited, it is usually most practical to leverage them as much as possible by selecting multiple applications that can share the use of the same resources—a process described often in this book as *leveraging resources*. Here are several examples:

- Connectivity among hospitals and doctors' offices would permit exchange of accounting and demographic information, clinical information such as results reporting, and consultations between doctors.

- Mechanisms for communicating with the population can be used for health assessment, for education, for public service bulletins, or to give or obtain patient-specific information.

- Connectivity between doctors' offices/homes and the Internet alone offers substantial scope for education, communicating with geographically dispersed colleagues, and collaboration.

- Development of a population database can lead to a community data repository that has many uses in planning, research, and education.

Leveraging resources is a key approach to maximizing the cost-effectiveness of any CHIN. If the ability to do so is not recognized, then the CHIN will be undervalued and undersold to potential CHIN supporters and participants. Several scenarios that use leveraged resources are described in Chapter 9, The Unifying CHIN. Because understanding these examples and applying them to real-life situations also requires a knowledge of several additional specific CHIN planning issues, these issues, which include medical informatics concerns, project management guidelines, and a number of technology-based topics such as security and the Internet, are reviewed first in Chapters 7 and 8.

Reference

Bazzoli, F. 1996. "Purchasers Push California CHIN." *Health Data Management* 4 (11): 50.

CHAPTER *7*

INFORMATION-BASED PLANNING CONCEPTS

Unless a community's healthcare stakeholders have worked together successfully in the past (as in the case of the Dayton,
Ohio, CHIN formed under the umbrella of the Greater Dayton Area
Hospital Association), community CHIN organizers need to take
the time to plan, learn, and adjust to the implications and impact
(Bazzoli 1996). Introducing a CHIN is really about introducing
change, so communities contemplating a CHIN need to temper their
expectations with the understanding that value will come from the
willingness to invest time, effort, and money in a smooth, welcomed
transition.

Thus far, the focus of this book has been on a fundamental source
of CHIN problems: understanding the potential value of the CHIN
and the CHINs' means of achieving that value for the community
and its healthcare enterprises. Healthcare executives should be aware
that other opportunities exist for misunderstanding and misstepping
in the planning phase, and that enterprises can guard against them.
This and the next chapter review several additional practical aspects
of planning that are intended as pointers for healthcare executives
who want to exercise further caution. In this chapter, the first focus
is on issues related to shared patient records, including quality,
identification, security, and the management of information. The
focus then shifts to information models for CHINs, moving from the
most basic of CHINs that provide only telecommunications services
to the most sophisticated models, those that are tightly integrated
into the healthcare system.

SHARING PATIENT RECORDS

Issues related to sharing patient records with other community enterprises are among the most contentious for healthcare executives. Earlier chapters described numerous ways to initiate a CHIN without the need to share individually identified patient records. Several such projects shown were in the goal-directed arenas of wellness, access, and improved quality of care. Inevitably, though, if the CHIN is to reach even a small part of its potential, sharing clinical information in patient records, either individually or for common purposes, will be necessary.

Already, most CHINs are helping enterprises to share clinical information when they send test results or discharge summaries to physicians' offices electronically. In that case, newly recorded data items, which presumably have been verified, are shared at about the same time they first enter the record. Sharing more complete patient records, full of historical information, is more than just a matter of transmitting data, however. Several of the complicating issues are listed here and discussed below:

- information quality;
- information identification;
- information security; and
- network management.

Information Quality

Quality discussions today center on the quality of care provided by institutions and larger enterprises. Since highly aggregated patient information is used to make those assessments, the quality of individual patient records, and of the individual data items in them, has not been a key issue.

When one provider shares an individual record with another who is treating the same patient at a different location, however, the second provider must be able to rely on the record as a basis for diagnosis and treatment. CHIN management must work with information suppliers to ensure that that is the case. For example, a clinic physician may need the patient's hospital records during a follow-up visit or the record of a trip to the emergency room of another hospital. In both cases, the first provider must do more than guarantee the correctness of individual data items. It must take responsibility as well for the completeness and accuracy of the entire portion of the record under its control. For completeness, all pertinent information must be transmitted. For accuracy, the temporal relationships of the data must be preserved and free from error.

Information Identification

Patient misidentification can have serious medical and financial consequences. As institutions increasingly are sharing records, whether within an enterprise composed of many institutions, or external to the enterprise, information identification has become an issue. Two aspects of record identification are important: identification of patient or member and the linking of multiple records for the same patient (Duncan 1996).

Patient identification

When a patient seeks treatment, his or her identity needs to be verified so that the correct medical records can be referenced. While this has always been the case, the problem is magnified today, since patients are seen routinely at multiple locations throughout the community. Health plans where this is a particular problem may already be using a *biometric identifier* such as a fingerprint, voice print, photograph, or retinal scan. In a community where patient affiliations with providers and health plans are shifting constantly, or where the population is mobile, it might make sense to consider a community-wide biometric identifier as part of the CHIN infrastructure.

Linkage of multiple records

A specific patient's medical records may reside in several hospitals, clinics, and physicians' offices throughout a community, as part of the continuum of care for which shared information is essential. Increasingly, enterprises are using information technology to create a centrally located link, or common patient directory called a *Master Patient Index* to associate a patient's multiple records with each other.

Where patient populations are shifting among community providers, CHIN participants need to create a Community MPI (CMPI) to locate a patient's records regardless of provider or plan. The CMPI would contain a unique community identifier, the location and identifier for each of the patient's medical records, possibly a biometric identifier, and selected personal and demographic information about the patient. The unique number identifier, which can be randomly generated, typically is used to link record fragments and not to identify the patient as a biometric identifier would. The Social Security number is a popular identifier, but as a record link it has fallen into disfavor, because Social Security numbers are not unique. Furthermore, they are used so widely in non-healthcare databases that their further use for healthcare constitutes a real threat to patient privacy when records are available electronically.

The initial task of matching and linking all of a patient's records through the CMPI can be daunting when multiplied by thousands, and perhaps tens of thousands, of people in the community. Software called *matching programs* enables the computer to help with this task.

Information Security

Three closely related terms are important to this discussion: privacy, confidentiality, and security. They are differentiated below.

- *Privacy* of information is the ability of an individual to control the use and dissemination of information that relates to himself or herself.
- *Confidentiality* is a tool for protecting privacy, because information designated as confidential requires strict controls on disclosure and access.
- *Security* includes all measures taken to safeguard a system and the information it contains or transmits, including measures to protect confidentiality (Electronic Frontier Foundation 1994).

Patient privacy

The issue of *patient privacy,* or the right of the patient to determine who shall have access to which information in his or her medical record, is at the top of the national healthcare agenda in Congress. Whereas information privacy has always been important to patients, information technology does provide new ways to violate it. Although privacy is a policy issue rather than a technical one, CHINs will still be responsible for treating patient records as confidential when they begin helping to share records.

CHIN developers will find that patients not only do not want their medical information disclosed or discovered, but they also do not want their appointments or billing information known, so providing confidentiality to protect patient privacy will not be an option. It is not enough that an enterprise tries to pass the risk to patients by having them sign statements allowing their records to be placed on the CHIN. Instead, CHIN developers must work with information suppliers and users to adopt a comprehensive and sensible security policy (Barrows and Clayton 1996).

End-to-end security

Traditional notions of security for an enterprise's health information network must expand to protect a CHIN adequately. The two key aspects of CHIN security are preserving confidentiality and assuring the physical integrity of the CHIN. Every CHIN should create and regularly test and update an end-to-end security plan encompassing all foreseeable security threats to the CHIN mission.

Breaches of security have many faces. They can be due to human error caused by an overly tired professional or by deliberate human mischief such as the work of hackers who take pleasure in violating the security of systems. Breaches can also take the form of a system failure, such as one that occurs when a piece of hardware breaks down or when an accident such as a fire damages equipment, software, and files. They can be relatively minor, such as a power outage during a storm, or devastating as in a natural disaster such as an earthquake. Each of these must be anticipated and prepared for to the extent possible.

The following sections describe specific breaches of security and the remedies available for their prevention, mitigation, or both.

Breaches of Confidentiality. Breaches of confidentiality today occur most commonly within the information supplier or user enterprise. The main sources are

- human error, such as occurs when the terminal with a patient record on the screen is left unattended, printouts are abandoned in the wastebasket, or test results are transmitted in error to the wrong doctor's office;

- legitimate users who access information they have no need to see, out of curiosity or with the intention of personal or financial gain; and

- outsiders who want information for personal reasons or financial gain, who want to do harm to a patient or the institution, or who just like a challenge.

Information supplier and user institutions can combat these kinds of security breaches with a mixture of organizational and technical mechanisms. Organizational practices include adoption of strict confidentiality policies combined with in-house training and even punitive measures. Technical safeguards include employing levels and types of access restricted by class of user, or even restricted to individual users; user authentication; and audit trails. User authentication in particular has been carried out in the past with a user ID number and a password that presumably only the user knows. Much more sophisticated techniques are available now, such as incorporating not only something only the user knows but also something only the user has, such as a "smart card" that can be read by an authorized terminal.

The biggest threat to patient privacy may come from the widespread dissemination of information throughout the healthcare system. Many groups in healthcare, including payors, oversight organizations, pharmaceutical companies, and equipment suppliers, collect large amounts of patient-identified information for legitimate purposes such as quality assessment or product improvement and marketing. No safeguards exist, however, to prevent further intended or unintended distribution and use, including perhaps even undesirable use from the patient's point of view. For example, self-insured employers collect patient information to monitor benefits programs and detect fraud. But there is nothing to prevent the employer from further using the information as the basis for denying promotions or even further employment.

Requiring that confidentiality be provided by non–care delivery organizations that possess patient information would require legislative or regulatory action. It is something CHIN participants should definitely consider supporting or even initiating, because the real value of the CHIN will depend increasingly on appropriate reuse of information from medical records to improve the healthcare system.

The foregoing discussion on security assumes that the CHIN is developed as a private network with restricted access. When a CHIN incorporates, or is connected to, the Internet, special security considerations arise. These are discussed in the section on the Internet and intranets in Chapter 8.

Physical Security of the CHIN.   The reliance on health information networks by healthcare enterprises is growing rapidly. CHIN developers need to recognize that patient care must continue even when the network is compromised. Further, if the CHIN is sufficiently mature as an integral part of many community healthcare projects, valuable project data and analyses may be threatened. Thus, the many and diverse connections made by CHINs dictate the need for careful attention to maintaining the physical integrity of the network, including protection against operational failures and provision for disaster recovery.

CHIN developers must consider the use of back-up power supplies and redundant hardware, so that when one component fails, another with the same functionality is already a part of the system and ready to do its job. Maintenance of backup for system and application software and databases must be planned to minimize the time lost in the event of failure.

Because problems are inevitable, developers need to work with CHIN enterprises to create an operating plan for information flow during periods when the system is not available. In the event of a major catastrophe, the CHIN may need to have in place a plan for operating at a different site for an extended period of time.

National Academy of Sciences Recommendations.   The National Academy of Sciences recently issued a highly readable and valuable report titled "For the Record: Protecting Electronic Health Information." It contains detailed explanations of threats to patient privacy and to the security of health information networks, and it makes extensive recommendations for organizational and technical security practices and procedures (Committee on Maintaining Privacy and Security for Health Care Applications on the National Information Infrastructure 1997).

Network Management

Sharing patient records adds layers of complexity for CHINs to manage. The definition of a medical record has been broadened by the continuum of care concept to include any medical record for a patient, no matter where in the community it may have been generated or stored. Some scholars would include any information about the patient in the new medical record, whether or not it was contained in the traditional medical record. In that case, additional types of information, such as demographic, social, employment, or academic data, all are considered to be relevant to a person's total well-being. Thus, the patient record (or member or citizen record) is a collection of record fragments unified by the CMPI.

The CMPI is itself a tool for the management of network complexity. Other management tools include capabilities for authorization, verification, routing, coping with simultaneous access, capacity management, audit, and accounting. Two additional important topics that relate to managing such a record are Central Data Repositories (CDRs) and brokering, both discussed below.

Central data repositories

A CDR is a serious option for sharing patient records. It may be a single database, or it may be composed of several smaller, related databases. For instance, a CDR might contain demographic and claims data for a community population. A separate CDR might contain patient data from the wellness educational program. The CMPI would provide a link between the demographic and claims data and the wellness data. The defining features of a CDR are that its records have more than one institutional source or more than one user organization can access them, or both. Several rationales for one or more CDRs are explored in Chapter 9.

Most CHIN participants think in terms of keeping the medical records they generate in-house. In some cases, however, it may be more practical to share a common database for at least some aspects of patient records. This could be instead of, or in addition to, the patient record database kept with the enterprise. Healthcare executives must keep in mind that the CDR only needs to contain portions of those records. The enterprise needs to share only what is agreed on to reach specific goals.

An option related to data repositories is whether to store a patient record as an optical image of pages in the record (like photographs or microfilms), or as digitized information that can be moved, abstracted, compiled, and analyzed. Optical images are replacing historical paper records at many institutions, and they are economical in cost and use of space. However, the records stored as optical images cannot be used in the future as electronic databases for research, education, and policy. They have the same disadvantages as paper records in that a researcher needs to go through the record visually to find needed information. The compromise would be to store old records as optical images, but begin putting new records, or new information for existing records, in an interactive database.

Brokering, or rules for CHINs

A rule book would be needed to guide the management of complex information through a CHIN. The concept of *brokering* has been defined as the establishment and application of just such a "rule book." It would cover such matters as the content, format, source, destination, route, timing, duration, and conditions for use of each piece of information. The brokering functions would obtain guidance from sources such as laws, regulations, contracts, memoranda of understanding, community standards, and common sense. CHIN participants clearly need to collaborate on the brokering function and establish standards in each area.

INFORMATION MODELS

This topic goes to the heart of whether a CHIN is a passive tool for telecommunications or whether it can in fact play a larger role in community health. It concerns whether the real task of a CHIN is to automate existing processes or to facilitate positive change in healthcare, even to the point of acting as a transforming agent. To the extent that different stakeholders hold different views, arriving at a common mission statement, goals, or even capabilities requires an exploration of this topic. Four models are discussed:

1. basic services information model;
2. value-added services information model;
3. value-added service provider information model; and
4. fully integrated information model.

The Basic Services Information Model

If the CHIN functions simply as a communications utility that is indifferent to, and not responsible for, the nature of the information it transmits, then it is providing *basic services* and leaving the burden of deciding what to do with the CHIN and the development and control of applications to individual participants. Typical basic services functions of network management that would be common to any approach include correct routing of the right information to the right place at the right time in a secure manner, confirmation that this has been done, provision of a transaction audit trail and other security measures, and a billing process for its own services. The more deeply the CHIN becomes involved in managing clinical information and applications, the more complex its basic functions become.

The Value-Added Services Information Model

If a CHIN provides *value-added services*, it actually processes information, adding value to it before or during transmission. As its applications become more complex, the CHIN can accept responsibility for at least these additional value-added services:

- verifying, encoding, collating, summarizing, merging, formatting, and analyzing information;

- implementing a complex array of security measures;

- managing, updating, maintaining, and purging one or more master indexes or data repositories; and

- maintaining, updating, and ensuring compliance with all of the laws, regulations, contracts, and standards that apply to the CHIN.

Community information service centers (CISCs) attached to the CHIN would perform these value-added services. Figure 7.1 shows a conceptual community information flow model for a CHIN. Note that any participant on the CHIN can be a source of information or a user, or both, and that the CISCs communicate over the CHIN with users and sources of information as well as with each other. Examples of service centers might be a central data repository, a statistical service center that performs analyses of information in a data repository, or a library that researches and fulfills requests for information held external to the CHIN.

The Value-Added Service
Provider Information Model

A more sophisticated addition is an information model that also relies on expert services attached to, but not a part of, the CHIN. These expert services would be supplied by *value-added service providers* (VSPs). VSPs would be incorporated when services require a level of expertise beyond those typical of a CHIN and its participants. Several examples of a VSP follow:

Figure 7.1 Value-Added Services Information Model

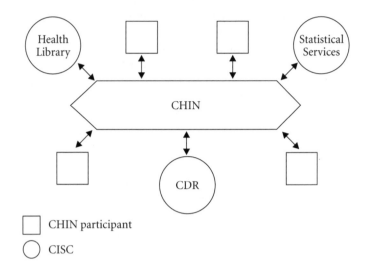

- A VSP with expertise in a clinical arena could direct all phases of a quality assessment program involving multiple providers.
- A disease management firm could deliver part of its services and share medical records with providers over the CHIN.
- A VSP with expertise in a skill arena such as education could develop, deliver, and evaluate wellness programs in the community.
- A VSP with marketing expertise could track consumer use of resources for community enterprise marketing purposes.

The CHIN could contract for the services of the VSP. Alternatively, groups or individual enterprises, or other stakeholders such as government agencies, could contract for such services. Furthermore, any of these could also offer VSP services over the CHIN. Figure 7.2 augments the basic CHIN information flow model to show that the relationship of a VSP to the other CHIN elements is indistinguishable from that of the CHIN elements themselves.

The Fully Integrated Information Model

In the *fully integrated information model*, the information system becomes the healthcare system, integrated as tightly and inseparably into the system as the physicians and patients themselves. All community stakeholders, including every provider, payor, consumer, agency, and school, are connected to the network, and all rely on

Figure 7.2   Value-Added Service Provider Information Model

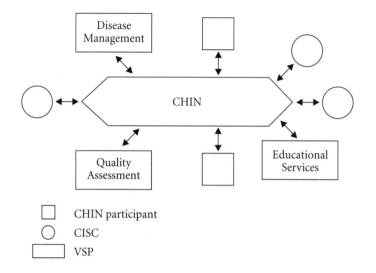

the network for healthcare communication. Each CHIN player has so many roles that distinctions are blurred and role definitions like those used in other information models have become meaningless. All but individual patient-identified or proprietary information flows freely, as though the CHIN were an interactive and enhanced library. Although this model requires a high degree of standardization and reliance, perhaps like that achieved for the automobile where we risk our lives daily, it can be achieved. The fully integrated information model is the subject of much of Chapter 8.

The choice among these four models, or any of many possible variations of them, depends on the goals of the network, with consideration given to the intentions and capabilities of the individual and organized stakeholders; the extent to which network functions are mandated by, for example, state government; and the resources available. Information technology has matured to the point where making the technology available is the least complicated part of a CHIN project. The challenge lies in how the CHIN is used, as demonstrated by the diversity of the information models.

References

Barrows, Jr., R. C., and P. D. Clayton. 1996. "Privacy, Confidentiality, and Electronic Medical Records." *Journal of the American Medical Informatics Association* 3 (2): 138–48.

Bazzoli, F. 1996. "Dayton Exemplifies the 'C' in CHIN." *Health Data Management* 4 (11): 54.

Committee on Maintaining Privacy and Security for Health Care Applications of the National Information Infrastructure. 1997. *For the Record: Protecting Electronic Health Information.* Washington, DC: National Academy Press.

Duncan, K. A. 1996. "ID Ideas: Patient Indexing Strategies for the New Continuum of Care." COMNET Society Journal 2 (1): 26–44.

Electronic Frontier Foundation Privacy and Technology Project. 1994. *Primer on Privacy.* Seattle, WA: Foundation for Health Care Quality.

CHAPTER 8

PLANNING THE CHIN INFRASTRUCTURE

This chapter continues to review other key aspects of planning the CHIN infrastructure, as a basis for discussions of the unifying CHIN in Chapter 9. We review the essentials for top-level planning as the first step in project management. The technology topics then presented are network design options, telecommunications, and the Internet and intranets.

PROJECT MANAGEMENT

For a highly complex project such as a CHIN to succeed, several ingredients must be present without fail. These key topics are strategic planning, realistic expectations, and knowledgeable leadership.

Strategic Planning

Several of the biggest tasks in strategic planning, and also the source of some of the most burdensome problems later, include establishing the mission, conducting due diligence, and exercising scope control. Elaboration of each of these follows.

Establishing the mission

This section pulls together the several aspects of mission discussed in several earlier chapters. The CHIN mission needs to be firmly imbedded in the mission of the system it serves. That is, the perspective should be, "Here are my goals; how can a CHIN help to meet them?" rather than, "Here is a CHIN; what should it do?"

Further, the mission and goal statements need to be endorsed by all stakeholders. The specific mission should be one that every participant agrees is important and is committed to fulfilling. In each case, the interests of all involved parties must be recognized and served, demonstrating the crucial factor, *alignment of mission*, which is the precursor to congruence of goals.

Participants enter into CHIN agreements for a staggering variety of reasons. To encompass all potential players, CHIN agreements are often written with a general, even idealistic, mission or goal statement. As time goes by, in the absence of focus on any common goal, each participant's sense of mission crystallizes as a personal mission. When the CHIN needs more resources or effort from its contributors, these new demands are evaluated in terms of progress toward the personal mission in each case—and are often found wanting.

A common misconception is that the vague goals, when achieved, will be global enough to include each personal goal. For instance, many CHINs were initiated for the purpose of putting a network in place, with no particular healthcare purpose in mind. The theory was that owners/stakeholders could use the capability for any legitimate purpose. When such a CHIN was constructed, it did not do anything useful, and major unanticipated costs and effort had to be incurred before it could.

While healthcare executives should of course consider the cost/benefit of CHIN participation, it is clear from the foregoing assertions that personal goals for the CHIN for improving one's own enterprise profitability at the expense of other participants is counterproductive. CHINs imply information sharing for common purposes. It is quite possible, however, to use CHINs and other forms of HINs to improve one's own position. For example, the cooperative development of patient education programs is a common goal, but how effectively each contributor uses the programs is a matter of individual initiative.

Due diligence

As an enterprise investment, a CHIN project should be subject to the same cautious scrutiny as any other investment of similar size and risk. That scrutiny is called *due diligence*, which is the obligation of planners to gain a thorough understanding of a project's goals, resources, constraints, and risks prior to launch. CHIN planners should undertake due diligence both on behalf of the CHIN and on behalf of the enterprises they represent. The critical questions are these:

• Does the project enhance the enterprise mission, community mission, or both for healthcare?

- Is the leadership competent, respected, and trustworthy?
- Are the plans credible and goal directed?

Before these assessments can be made, it is usually necessary to study the demographics and character of the community, its healthcare system, its information flow dynamics and needs, the information technology and project management expertise in the community, and sources of funding and technology. Healthcare executives should ask themselves if they are willing to commit resources needed to accomplish the CHIN, and they should ask their potential partners the same question. Attitudes, motivation, and other subtle factors concerning the people and enterprises involved might also affect success.

The same questions need to be asked, whether a CHIN is just beginning or is planning to expand. A conservative CHIN, flush with the success of its initial program, must rely on due diligence and scope control as much in the second round as in the first.

Scope control

The uses of information technology in healthcare are practically limitless. It is appropriate for knowledgeable planners to envision the unfolding of a CHIN's scope into the future, to include not only all possible interlocking and integrated capabilities, but also to reach beyond the community to the state or even the nation. In fact, if CHIN goals are too limited, opportunities may be missed. If the full potential of the CHIN is understood, its assets can be leveraged across several arenas during implementation planning. Further, a diverse scope helps a CHIN serve a more diverse group of stakeholders.

On the other hand, global goals may overwhelm potential partners. In reality, simply developing a significant capability in a few areas involving a limited number of the community stakeholders is a task that will probably occupy CHIN initiators for several years. A timeline for achieving various functionalities helps to clarify scope.

Realistic Expectations

As the CHIN movement was gathering steam, some very good models existed, notably the Wisconsin Health Information Network and several implementations of the RWJ Foundation-funded CHMIS program mentioned earlier. Even though these early CHINs worked well, the reasons for their successes were not well understood. Potential developers hoping to emulate their success failed to perceive the complexity of the task and the need for strategic planning, and participants did not foresee the extent of the resources, creativity, disruption, change, and commitment their participation would require. The aspiring CHINs overestimated the capabilities of information technology while they underestimated the demands that would be placed on them. Ultimately, the payoff for participation appeared so far removed in time from the cost and effort that the venture became impossible to justify. No other CHIN need repeat this discouraging process.

Knowledgeable Leadership

Charisma, political and oratorical skills, and commitment to the rightness of the CHIN characterize CHIN leaders. But they need more than these qualities for commanding enthusiasm, belief, support, and loyalty. A CHIN leader must be prepared to take end-to-end responsibility for the functional design and impact of the CHIN.

The complexity of CHIN initiatives cannot be overestimated. CHIN leaders must also have knowledge, or at least understanding, of

- healthcare system dynamics, especially those of the clinical care system;
- information technology network concepts and function;
- the sociology of healthcare and the population it serves; and
- issues at the interfaces of healthcare, information technology, and society.

Several of these issues are practical, such as the lack of data and interface standards or the reliability of telecommunications networks. Others, such as confidentiality of patient data or the impact of networking on job functions, are sociological.

TECHNOLOGY TOPICS

Fortunately for CHIN initiators, available information technology can meet the needs of almost any kind of CHIN. Technical choices and solutions at the cutting edge are relatively straightforward. On the other hand, CHIN capabilities can be built on a variety of existing technology platforms (bases) to match the needs, resources, and constraints of the community. However, some technology options remain controversial, and it is important that healthcare executives understand their implications. Three key technology topics are the subject of the next sections:

1. network architecture options;
2. telecommunications options; and
3. the Internet versus intranets.

Network Design Options

Both centralized and distributed networking approaches have been used for CHINs. A centralized networking approach is considered by many to be a thing of the past. While it is true that new systems are being designed around a distributed approach, satisfactory CHINs can be established with either one.

For the *centralized networking approach*, the CHIN would use a single large computer system, or a mainframe system, to store information, provide services, and carry out the CHIN functions. Information sources, users, CISCs, and VSPs throughout the community would be connected to the mainframe by telecommunications technology. A CHIN might use this approach to take advantage, for instance, of a large mainframe computer system already available in a hospital or at an insurance company's facilities. A vendor might propose this approach, making available a single large regional facility to which providers could subscribe.

When new information technology systems are planned, CHINs more typically would plan to use the *distributed networking approach* such as client (user) server architecture. A server is a special-purpose computer on the network. For instance, a server that manages the Master Patient Index would be different from the server that manages the educational programs or the quality information.

The CHIN functions and the information and services available for CHIN users would be distributed among servers connected by a telecommunications device called a *wide area network* (WAN). Because the users are also connected to the WAN, they have access to the information and services provided by all the servers.

Figure 8.1 shows a schematic contrasting the architecture of the two approaches. Regardless of the technical platform, the information flow models are the same in either case from the point of view of the user. For instance, the Master Patient Index and the Central Data Repository would function in the same way, from the user's point of view. Thus a healthcare professional using the network should not be able to detect the difference between the two approaches.

A client server system at least has the advantage of greater flexibility when it comes to adding CHIN capabilities and functions. New servers are added to carry out new functions over the same telecommunications WAN.

Some communities may want to initiate their CHIN by using an available mainframe system, and then later migrating to a client server system. It is quite possible to do so. When the client server system is added to the CHIN, the mainframe simply becomes a server in the

Figure 8.1 Contrasting Network Approaches

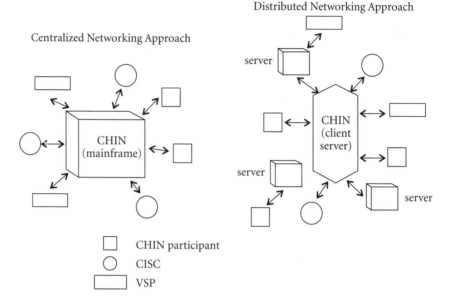

Centralized Networking Approach

Distributed Networking Approach

☐ CHIN participant
○ CISC
▭ VSP

new network and continues to perform its functions. Users who were previously connected directly to the mainframe would now access the mainframe through the client server network. The CHIN would then be further developed and extended by adding new functions and servers directly to the network instead of to the mainframe.

Telecommunications Capabilities

Almost all CHINs, and indeed almost all health information networks, transmit information over telephone lines. These lines may be public, but usually they are leased and dedicated to the CHIN, and therefore are more secure. In any case, data transmission is typically at speeds so great that a person using a computer terminal perceives the transaction time to be only a split second.

CHINs need to transmit not only data and voice, but also information-dense materials such as high-quality video or x-ray images. For telemedicine applications, in particular, where diagnostic-quality video images must be transmitted over a period of time, CHINs are pushing the limits of communications capacity. While conventional modems, which allow individual computer terminals to communicate over the CHIN, have a practical limit of 56 kilobits per second, high-speed communications technology is available in the range of 10–100 megabits (equivalent to millions of words) per second.

Telecommunications offerings are getting faster, and future options will include not only standard phone lines but also wireless and cable. The telecommunications industry is heavily regulated, but healthcare may expect some regulatory relief, especially for telemedicine applications. CHIN telecommunications strategies should be flexible, so that they can take ready advantage of both technical and political opportunities. Developers should be aware of the various industry *communications standards* and the need for compatibility among all network components.

The Internet and Intranets

The Internet and intranets offer sophisticated networking approaches and capabilities of high potential for healthcare. They are described and contrasted below, and their relevance to CHINs is discussed.

The Internet

The *Internet* is a wonderful, amorphous network that facilitates global location and sharing of information of every sort, including extensive healthcare information for professionals and consumers. Several popular features that are relevant to CHINs are electronic mail, information browsing, transporting work files, and collaborative work, such as occurs in the Genome Project.

Like the healthcare system, the Internet is a system where the individual elements do what they do more or less by common consent. Again like the healthcare system, there is no organizational infrastructure, no policymaking body, no planning, and no central management or coordination. In short, no one is in charge.

Although the Internet appears to be a recent phenomenon, development of the precursor network to the Internet began in the late1960s under the auspices of the Department of Defense (Hafner and Lyon 1996). The original network, called the Arpanet, was used primarily by academic and scientific institutions for research. The Arpanet grew and evolved over the years to become part of the massive interconnection of several networks—dubbed the Internet—that we use today (Salus 1995).

The Internet was popular from the beginning because it was so easy to make information available and so easy to use. Unfortunately for the healthcare community, it is also unreliable and its security is easily breached. Because it is a public network, the Internet is susceptible to hackers who can break through network security (usually consisting of an ID and password), destroying user files and systems, violating the privacy of Internet users by "stealing" personal information, or corrupting information available on the Internet. Even worse from a healthcare point of view, the Internet is highly vulnerable to service failures due to power or phone line outages, physical damage to facilities, and even poor planning by service providers. Consider these recent news stories and the potential for harm to healthcare enterprises dependent on the Internet for availability of patient records:

- A hacker gathered 100,000 credit card numbers and enough information to use them by working his way into a San Diego–based Internet provider. The information belonged to a dozen companies selling products over the network. He accessed the provider through an account at the University of California at San Diego (FBI Nabs Major Hacker 1997).

- A programming error at Networking Solutions, Inc., the Virginia-based organization responsible for assigning most electronic addresses on the Internet, caused millions of electronic mail messages from around the world to be returned to their senders as undeliverable (Markoff 1997).

- When rats got into an electrical transformer at Stanford University, the entire San Francisco Bay Area regional node of the Internet was out of service for 24 hours, affecting millions of Internet users.

In other examples, America Online, a company that links individuals and businesses to the Internet, recently changed its billing from hourly charges to a flat monthly fee. The company was so swamped by the increase in attempted use that all of its Internet connections were out of service for days. Outages of electrical power and the telephone system—both of which are part of the essential infrastructure for the Internet—have disrupted Internet service repeatedly and will continue to do so.

Some healthcare organizations, most notably academic institutions, are investigating the feasibility of transmitting or otherwise making patient-specific information selectively available over the Internet. However, in addition to the day-to-day potential for Internet failure, the potential for security breaches, and the lack of a reliable infrastructure, some experts believe that the Internet is also operating at near its transmission capacity. For these very good reasons CHIN planners should not expect to rely on the Internet in the next several years as a way to make patient records available.

As Internet security, reliability, and organizational problems become resolved over time, CHIN long-range planning should definitely include using it. Advances in cryptography are already facilitating electronic commerce over the Internet, and cryptography will solve some of the security problems for electronic patient records as well. However, electronic commerce does not require the same level of reliability as patient records would. For instance, Internet credit card orders can tolerate transaction delays of hours or even days, but that level of service would not be acceptable to clinicians who might need a patient record immediately.

The Internet can be an excellent way to communicate nonpatient information. Many healthcare enterprises use the Internet as a way of making factual information available to the community and beyond. For example, they may make available for any reader a range of information about their hospitals, doctors, specialties, and training programs. They may list job openings and public telephone numbers. They may even provide educational materials and disease-specific databases pointing to references and resources.

None of this information is patient specific or even about patients. If any of the information were temporarily unavailable because the Internet were unavailable, no harm would be done. Even if the information were destroyed, the information could easily be replaced. CHIN planners who want to incorporate the Internet into their activities should consider these kinds of noncritical capabilities.

Internet II, a new network that will be 100 times faster than the current Internet, is being planned. It is being developed primarily by and for academic and research institutions, because researchers believe that the Internet is too congested for these organizations' needs. Internet II should also be available to healthcare for education and research.

The next section discusses an excellent community alternative to the Internet.

Intranets

Intranets are private networks belonging to enterprises that use the same protocols and technologies as the Internet (Siwicki 1996). Geographically dispersed enterprises use intranets to facilitate information sharing within the enterprise. The intranet concept would be an ideal option for a CHIN. It has the advantage of the Internet's low cost and ease of use without as much scope for outsider security threats and system failures.

An intranet could be incorporated into a CHIN for information dissemination to professionals and consumers in much the same way that was described for the Internet. In fact, intranets are regarded by many as a new publishing medium for such internal documents as policy manuals, directories, and instruction manuals. In addition to publishing complete provider and plan information, extensive community-specific healthcare information such as resource and referral services databases, local classes, and interactive educational materials could be made available over the CHIN. Such materials are easily updated and always available.

An intranet is relatively easy to install and use, but since any computer on the intranet can become a server providing information to others, insider security breaches may become a problem. The CHIN security plan must include this as a heightened risk. It is important to note that an intranet is not a substitute for a health information network like a CHIN since, like the Internet, an intranet currently does not have much capability beyond information sharing. Complex clinical applications are beyond its scope.

Linking intranets and the Internet

CHIN intranet users, like those in any enterprise, would still want access to the full range of global Internet capabilities. When the intranet interfaces with the Internet, the intranet is once again vulnerable to intruders. Intranets can be protected by establishing a single computer as a gateway between the intranet and the Internet and placing a software *firewall* between the two. The firewall monitors traffic from the Internet and controls outsider access to systems inside on the intranet.

A large CHIN with technology-sophisticated participants would no doubt have several servers that are also connected directly to the Internet. These servers can also be protected from intruders by special software that monitors and controls access.

Where patient records on the Internet are involved, the National Academy of Sciences report on privacy and security cited in Chapter 7 strongly recommends such extra security precautions as firewalls. In addition they recommend that modern encryption techniques be used for all patient-related information, including that transmitted by e-mail (Committee on Maintaining Privacy and Security for Health Care Applications on the National Information Infrastructure 1997). This applies to any transmission outside the organizational boundary (a private intranet is considered to be inside the organization). In fact, they recommend that any enterprise that does not use cryptography for patient information should refrain from sharing patient records outside the enterprise. These security measures apply to communicating over any public network, such as a physician does when he or she dials a CHIN server over public phone lines from a computer at home. Public network communication would also require additional secure authorization methods.

Chapters 7 and 8 have reviewed an array of key concepts related to CHIN planning. These ranged from the information-based concepts of patient records-sharing, information security, and selection of a CHIN information model, to important aspects of project management for CHINs and consideration of technology options. These concepts, together with the value assessment and building block analyses, provide the groundwork for discussion of the unifying CHIN in the next chapter.

References

Committee on Maintaining Privacy and Security for Health Care Applications for the National Information Infrastructure. 1997. *For the Record: Protecting Electronic Health Information.* Washington, DC: National Academy Press.

"FBI Nabs Major Hacker." 1997. *San Francisco Chronicle* May 23, p. C1–2.

Hafner, K., and M. Lyon. 1996. *Where Wizards Stay Up Late.* New York: Simon and Schuster.

Markoff, J. 1997. "Snafu Snarls The Internet Worldwide." *San Francisco Chronicle* July 18, 1997, p. A1, A14.

Salus, P. H. 1995. *Casing the Net.* Reading, MA: Addison-Wesley.

Siwicki, B. 1996. "Intranets in Health Care." *Health Data Management* 4 (8): 36–47.

CHAPTER 9

THE UNIFYING CHIN

A CHIN has its greatest value when its assets are leveraged to meet the information needs of stakeholders across the healthcare spectrum. Too often, a single-purpose CHIN, using expensive information technology to replace existing functions, appears to be implementing change for the sake of change. Installing a single-purpose CHIN is like buying a car with only one gear or, worse, no steering wheel: it is useful for some purposes in the short term, perhaps, but too limiting to consider as a reason for long-term investment. A CHIN needs to do things that are new, things that help a community achieve in areas where achievement was previously not possible.

This chapter shows how a community can get more value out of its CHIN by taking advantage of opportunities to use community capabilities and CHIN building blocks repeatedly and for multiple purposes. First, several important community healthcare information cycles, or projects—all hypothetical—are described in terms of one or more of the information flow models presented in Chapter 7. These cycles are then used to demonstrate several advanced CHIN concepts. They show the interdependence of information needs and ways in which this interdependency can take advantage of CHIN capabilities. They also show the redundancy in health information flow that can be eliminated by the unifying CHIN.

THE COMMUNITY QUALITY
REVIEW PROJECT

Chapter 3 showed that there are many ways to view quality of care and many levels on which improved quality can be addressed. Each involves a cycle whereby clinician performance is measured to assess quality of care, but performance measures also serve as feedback for making targeted quality-improvement information available to clinicians. CHIN initiators who understand that clinicians need more guidance in their practices than is currently available can actually implement a measurably effective quality improvement program at the community level. A county medical society conceived and supported this quality improvement project. Consider this example from the point of view of a community primary care physician.

The Clinician's View

Dr. Addie Hurst turns to her office computer at the end of the day. She sees that the monthly Quality Review is available, so she enters her special code number and spends the next five minutes interacting with the computer program. The Quality Review this month first reviews for Dr. Hurst the community guidelines for managing the care of patients with asthma. The guidelines, which are suggestions rather than rules, are the product of a consensus of community physicians who are experts in the field. The computer program then shows a summary of community physician compliance with the asthma guidelines over the past six months, and it shows her individual compliance over that same period of time. Based on her performance, additional materials for review are suggested. These may be articles, literature reviews, or practice simulations, all of which are available from her office or home computer. Last month, the Quality Review focused on management of Type II diabetes; next month, the topic will be indications for cholesterol-lowering therapy.

Dr. Hurst always knows at least eight months in advance what the upcoming Quality Review schedule of topics will be, and she has the same advance access to the guidelines. The opportunity to review, followed by feedback on her subsequent performance, with a reinforcing opportunity to review again six months later, suits both her need for up-to-date information and her busy practice style. Whenever the guidelines are significantly updated, she receives an announcement by e-mail that she should review the guidelines again. Her participation is by subscription and entirely voluntary, although some community health plans and physician groups require participation.

The Quality Review Information Model

How is this simple feedback to Dr. Hurst achieved through the CHIN? We will use the CHIN information flow model with VSPs to analyze the project. Clearly, Dr. Hurst is the primary user. It is her behavior that the project hopes and expects to influence, with the community as a whole as the beneficiary when most physicians participate. Many other steps are needed to make this possible, however.

Information suppliers

Dr. Hurst is also an information source, or supplier. In her office she routinely uses one of several versions of a CPR approved by the Community Quality Review Project. With the CPR, it is easy for her to select and send patient information for evaluation. For this month's project, her assistant first submitted electronically the baseline information on all of Dr. Hurst's asthma patients. Then for the six-month period of the performance review, her assistant transmitted the encounter information for those patients as convenient. A computer program to do this automatically could be incorporated with the CPR.

Dr. Hurst's identity is not known to the Quality Review Project implementers. No one but she sees her results or otherwise passes judgment on her work. She submits and retrieves all information using only her code number. Her patients' identities are not known either; during a Quality Review cycle, she uses a temporary sequence number for each patient.

Dr. Hurst's colleague practicing in an adjacent office building, Dr. Carl Peterson, also subscribes to the Quality Review Project, but he does not have a computer-based patient record. He receives the guideline review and community-wide performance measures over his office computer like Dr. Hurst does. However, since Dr. Peterson must extract baseline and encounter information from his paper-based patient records, he only participates in one or two performance feedback cycles of particular interest to him each year.

Hospitals and other community providers are the second group of information suppliers. Payors require that utilization and outcome data from the hospitals where Dr. Hurst is on the staff be available electronically, and this information can also be used for the Quality Review Project as appropriate. For the current review on asthma, the frequency of Dr. Hurst's admissions for asthma is needed, but the admissions do not need to be tied to particular patients. In reviews where outcomes are needed for specific patients, an agency separate from the Quality Review implementers would use the community's Master Patient Index, or CMPI, to link the hospital records with the office encounter records and then strip the identifiers before sending them on to the Quality Review Project. That agency is a separate CHIN information service center, or CISC, that manages the CMPI.

Information service centers

The raw data for determining utilization and outcomes for all hospitals are maintained in a CDR. It is one of many linked databases maintained by the CHIN at a CISC. Because all hospitals must provide similar information for payors and purchasers for all their patient population, each hospital places a copy of agreed-upon portions of their patient records database, hospital-identified and doctor-identified but with patient identifiers removed, in a common CHIN CDR. The Quality Review Project is just one of many CHIN projects authorized to use selected portions of these data for sanctioned purposes.

Value-added service providers

The Quality Review Project requires tools and skills beyond those routinely available through the CHIN. First, hospital and clinic patient records need to be researched for topics where community physicians in general need more guidance than they apparently have now. A community clinical team then needs to collaborate on and gain general endorsement of the guidelines for the selected topics. Medical knowledge base experts need to select review materials and manage the development of the case simulations. Other experts need to custom design performance measures that are appropriate for each of the monthly review topics. Still others need to manage the entire process, including developing programs for delivering information to the clinicians. To accomplish all these steps, the CHIN has a contract with a VSP, Biometrics Unlimited, to design, implement, and manage the Quality Review Project for the community.

The information flow model for this project is shown in Figure 9.1. Note that it includes many CHIN enterprises such as plans, hospitals, and doctors' offices, as well as a CISC and the VSP.

Quality Review Project Summary

The Quality Review Project is conceptually simple and rewarding for physicians and the community without being intrusive. It respects the privacy of not only the patients, but also the physicians and hospitals. It is important to note, however, that such projects have nothing to do with competition. Their goals can only be achieved collaboratively. Not every physician and hospital need agree to participate, but certainly a critical mass must do so, in order to make a valid inference to community practices as a whole.

Of course, each enterprise or each payor could establish its own Quality Review Project, using just its own hospitals and physicians, but the duplication of effort and resources is needless at best. By

Figure 9.1 The Quality Review Project Information Flow

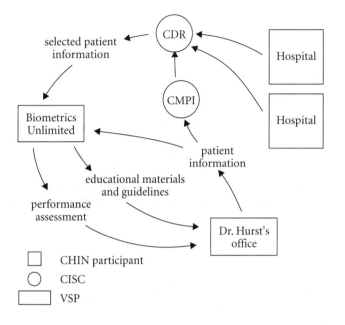

collaborating, all community enterprises can share in the communications facilities, the project development and management costs of the VSP, and the conceptualization and creativity needed at several points. Further, as noted in Chapter 3, purchasers, payors, and consumers should insist that enterprises demonstrably meet at least community standards of care rather than simply their own.

Leveraging the Project

It is difficult to consider even one community healthcare information cycle without observing the scope for leveraging CHIN and other information technology-related assets many times over. The office-based CPR and the hospital-based CPR would have many uses, both for internal management and for external reporting, consultation, and research. The Quality Review Project itself can be leveraged in larger communities. The processes can be applied to management of problems in virtually any medical specialty, as well as the primary care uses in this example. Some topics could even be leveraged by using them for multiple groups. For example, indications for cholesterol-lowering therapy would be a topic of interest to both primary care physicians and cardiologists.

THE COMMUNITY ENTERPRISE MARKETING PROJECT

Major healthcare enterprises' participation in their community's CHIN is all but essential for long-term CHIN value and success. At a minimum, the patient information they possess is an almost indispensable resource, and their commitment and expertise is invaluable. For such enterprises, competition is a prime concern, so this example of a marketing cycle should be of particular interest. The premise of this cycle is that enterprises need to collaborate in the information sphere in order to compete on the quality, convenience, and price of their product. In this cycle, community providers share performance information with payors, who in turn share administrative tools and financial information with providers. Consider this example from the point of view of Dallas Edward General Hospital and the Westminster Classic Health Plan.

The Hospital's View

Dallas Edward General is a medium-sized public hospital, one of several in a sprawling metropolitan area. Many of its staff physicians use several other community hospitals as well. Dallas General has contracts with several managed care plans, each of which has its own requirements for accountability regarding quality of care. Among these plans is the Westminster Classic, a small plan heavily subscribed to by local businesses. Besides the accountability Westminster itself requires of Dallas General, additional quality-related information requirements are imposed through Westminster by purchasers and accreditors.

Community CHIN initiators recognized that the purchasers and accreditors are substantially the same for all of the plans and hospitals, and so, therefore, were the information demands on all the hospitals. Consequently, CHIN initiators proposed a cooperative approach to meeting the information needs.

Annually, Dallas General prepares an extensive extract of its patient database and transmits it to a CDR at a CHIN information services center. All the other participating community hospitals do the same. The information is hospital-, plan-, and doctor-identified (and possibly purchaser-identified), but not patient-identified. The raw data are transmitted according to a detailed and complex brokering agreement among the community's plans, purchasers, and hospitals. The data are to be used for utilization and outcomes analysis.

A VSP named Hickory Acres Marketing, also acting in accordance with a brokering agreement, uses the information in the CHIN-controlled CDR to prepare utilization reports and outcome analyses.

Hickory Acres knows exactly which information, in what format, is needed for each purchaser, plan, and accreditor, and it prepares analyses, summaries, and reports accordingly. Reports are generated by plan, by hospital, and for the community as a whole and made available according to the brokering agreements.

The Health Plan's View

Westminster Classic incorporates the purchaser-specific analyses for its members into the reports it is making to current purchasers. It uses hospital-by-hospital analyses for presentations to potential purchasers. Selected information is used for marketing to the community. Westminster also uses the analyses to help meet accrediting bodies' requirements. In all cases, Westminster decides which information it wants to release and to whom.

To complete the marketing cycle, Dallas General receives information in exchange for its cooperation in supplying raw data. First, Hickory Acres supplies Dallas General with all of the information it is reporting about Dallas General and with communitywide summary information. The hospital uses this information in its accreditation process and for in-house management and quality improvement programs. Second, Dallas General has on-line access to Westminster's enrollment database, and also that of every plan with whom the hospital contracts. Each plan database contains a membership roster with member identification and benefit information. Each of Dallas General's staff physicians whose office computer is connected to the CHIN may also access the plan databases.

The Enterprise Marketing Information Model

In exemplary CHIN fashion, a variety of stakeholders meet their information needs while at the same time helping to meet the needs of others. Using the Enterprise Marketing cycle, the utilization and outcome analyses already required throughout the community are performed consistently and economically for all enterprises. Plans and hospitals have the analyses they need in support of quality assessment for marketing or accreditation purposes.

Dallas General is an information supplier when it originates information for the CHIN—in this case a portion of its patient database. It is also an information end-user of reports prepared by Hickory Acres and of the plan databases. Similarly, Westminster Classic is an information supplier of its membership database and a user of the VSP's reports. Physicians who access the plan membership databases are also information users.

Enterprise Marketing includes a CISC to manage and control access to the CDR containing the patient record extracts. It also includes the Hickory Acres Marketing VSP. The VSP helped to negotiate all the brokering agreements among all parties. It has ongoing responsibility for all analyses and reporting as well as for a system of quality control for its work.

It is worth noting that brokering agreements surround all elements of the cycle, covering everything from the quality of the information supplied to the content and timing of reports, to guidelines for updating and purging databases. Brokering agreements of various sorts apply to Dallas General, to Westminster Classic, Hickory Acres Marketing, and even elements of the CHIN itself, such as the information service centers that manage the CDR. Figure 9.2 shows the information flow for the Enterprise Marketing Project, including multiple plans and multiple hospitals.

The Enterprise Marketing Project Summary

Generating meaningful utilization and outcome analyses is a lot of work, not the least of which is deciding what information to collect and analyze. Reporting requirements are expected to grow more complex every year, but this is true whether the process is automated and whether it is achieved on an enterprise-by-enterprise basis or

Figure 9.2 The Enterprise Marketing Project Information Flow

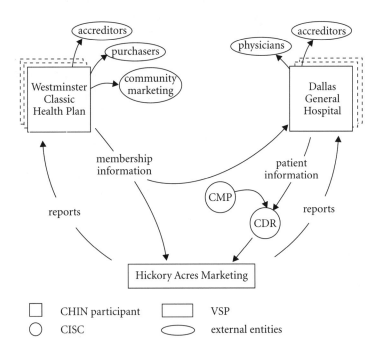

with a CHIN. With the Enterprise Marketing Project, however, once the decision is made about the analyses required, and the necessary information is transferred to a CHIN CDR, the work of Dallas General and Westminster is essentially done. To complete the cycle, access to Westminster Classic's member database and that of the other participating plans offers considerable administrative simplification and savings for hospitals and doctors.

Regardless of the number of plans, purchasers, and accreditors involved, the information is only collected and processed once by the enterprises. Information users get only the agreed-upon information. Analyses, reports, and summaries are prepared uniformly, so they are directly combinable by the plans and, for purchasers, comparable across hospitals and plans. In short, the Enterprise Marketing cycle is an example of a labor- and cost-saving process that improves the quality and value of essential information.

Leveraging the Project

The project's hallmark building block that can be leveraged for the future is the collaborative infrastructure established among the major community healthcare enterprises—primarily plans and hospitals. The (technically) simple CHIN capability demonstrated here only scratches the surface of the opportunities for collaboration. In this case, the enterprises have decided that evaluation science is not sufficiently advanced for hospital and plan comparisons by the public. However, just collaborative enterprise reuse of the database derived from patient records can lead to additional quality assurance studies. For instance, the hospitals and plans can use such studies as the basis for community, plan, or hospital quality improvement measures over and above those required by purchasers or accreditors.

The linkages created by this project can become part of, or lead to, a larger financial system that includes claims processing. Such a system can easily extend to physicians' offices, not only encompassing plan and financial information, but also allowing analysis of physician-patient encounter data.

THE MINING CARRYOVER PROJECT

Kaysburg is a former mining town in the Ohio River Valley. Because of its lovely setting, the area is enjoying a resurgence in popularity and population growth. The employees of several new light industries appreciate the easy semirural lifestyle combined with modern development. However, Dr. Jeff Roberts, director of the Kaysburg County Public Health Department, is concerned that the mining history of the area may pose a health threat to the growing community. Environmental testing has been inconclusive.

The Public Health Department's

Working with the Centers for Disease Control and Prevention in Atlanta, Dr. Roberts' staff has identified the most likely environmental threats. The possible resulting health problems are serious. He decides to establish the five-to-ten year Mining Carryover Project to monitor the levels of these problems in the community and then deal with them aggressively. If the level of health problems warrants, Dr. Roberts will apply for funding from the Federal Toxic Waste Cleanup Superfund.

To monitor the population for the relevant symptoms and diagnoses, Dr. Roberts needs to enlist the cooperation of Kaysburg's providers for data collection. He also needs to educate Kaysburg's physicians about what to look for and how to proceed with diagnosis and treatment planning.

Because of its recent rapid growth, much of the Kaysburg healthcare infrastructure is new, so implementation of health information networks is already widespread. Dr. Roberts spearheads the creation of a CHIN to which all the hospitals, clinics, and individual doctors offices in the county may connect. The project is so important to the survival of the community that it has broad community support and funding from outside the healthcare system, as well as within it.

Dr. Roberts contracts with Naples Clinical Decision Support Services, a VSP, to develop and manage the project on behalf of the Public Health Department. The project has four information components:

1. collecting problem-specific information from providers;
2. providing guidelines and other educational materials such as practice simulations for physicians;
3. evaluating results; and
4. incorporating the feedback into the data collection and education processes.

When Dr. Stephanie Marius, a community physician, encounters a patient with one of the targeted health problems, an extensive round of data collection is initiated. To make it as convenient as possible for her, Naples Services has designed a basic reporting form that the office or clinic staff may use. The form may be filled out manually and mailed in, but Dr. Marius has a CPR, so Naples Services provides software to extract the information directly from the CPR. The information goes directly to Naples Services for analysis.

Hospitals need to provide only diagnoses and outcomes for this project. Their staff may fill out forms manually, or the hospital may use the Naples software to extract the information directly from the CPR.

Naples Services also designs the guidelines and educational materials for the anticipated problems. These can be given to physicians in printed form, or they can be accessed over an office or home computer. For physicians with office computers, the guidelines also can be used interactively during a patient encounter.

Although participation in the project is voluntary during the early stages, virtually every primary care physician and specialist in Kaysburg County participates. If and when problems surface at a significant level, participation would be mandatory.

The Mining Carryover Information Model

The Mining Carryover Project demonstrates the information flow cycle of yet another dimension of healthcare, namely, public health. The primary beneficiary of the CHIN project is the entire community of Kaysburg. It is important to understand that the beneficiaries are not just individual citizens, but also the Kaysburg business community, which depends on a healthy environment for survival.

The information providers are the physicians and hospitals, and the Public Health Department through its VSP agent, Naples Clinical Decision Support Services. The information users are the physicians, who use the guidelines and educational programs, and the Public Health Department, which receives extensive amounts of data and analyses from Naples Services.

The information model incorporates Naples Services as a VSP. Naples Services maintains for analysis a problem-specific database drawn from hospital and physician input, whether manual or electronic. It uses the CISC that manages the CMPI to link the hospital and physician records. This project does not require a CDR. However, if one or more of the hospitals routinely places all or part of its patient record database in a CHIN CDR, then Naples Services can access that CISC for hospital data instead of asking the hospital directly for the data. Figure 9.3 shows the Mining Carryover Project information flow, including multiple hospitals and multiple doctors' offices.

The Mining Carryover Project Summary

The Kaysburg CHIN easily facilitates a public health project that is vital to the future well-being of the community. Because the CHIN provides a robust mechanism for information flow, the community's professional resources can be focused on the clinical problems rather than on the process. Of course, the greater the community's saturation with office computers and CPRs, the more valuable the CHIN becomes for this project.

Figure 9.3   The Mining Carryover Project Information Flow

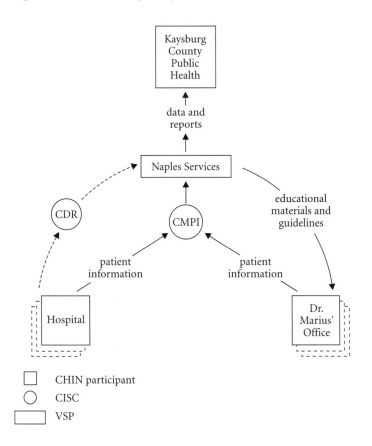

Leveraging the Pr◗

Once a public health monitoring system similar to the one designed for the Mining Carryover Project is in place, it is possible to correlate health problems with other community conditions in addition to environmental hazards. The research and development programs and tools prepared by Naples Services would be adaptable to new areas. For instance, social services available in the community, employment status, place of employment, and educational status may also affect health and health expectations. Such analyses could lead to preventive interventions and targeted physician education programs. Automatic tracking of traditional health indicators such as instances of infectious diseases is also possible where CPRs are available.

THE COMMUNITY WELLNESS
PROJECT REVISITED · · · · · · · · · · · · ·

Chapter 6 described a Community Wellness Project, whereby specific medical problems were tackled using an aggressive combination of community education and health status monitoring. The project is highly successful, and local businesses are enthusiastic. The hospitals have decided to work with CHIN director Dr. Nellie Simons to expand it to include additional appropriate medical problems. Various CHIN partners have been taking responsibility for parts of the project, but managing the information flow is so labor intensive that other arrangements will have to be made for the expanded project.

Expanding the CHIN for this project has three major steps:

1. First, Dr. Simons creates two CDRs. One is the existing and expanding population database. The other is made up of partial patient records from the hospitals. Each CDR is the responsibility of a CISC.

2. Since the Community Wellness Project is going to be a permanent capability, Dr. Simons contracts with a VSP, New-Way Health-care, to develop the new educational and evaluation materials and manage the project. The community clinical board that has been selecting the medical problems continues in that role and provides oversight.

3. Dr. Simons institutes new security measures. The population database, which heretofore has not necessarily contained person-specific information, needs to do so in the future. Because the CHIN will be delivering its educational materials and collecting its population evaluations over the Internet, special security measures are needed to prevent records in the population database from being accessed over the Internet.

The new CDR containing extracts of patient records will not be accessible over the Internet at all, and its location needs to be secured. At this point, only the hospitals can update it and only New-Way, the VSP, can read information in the database. These elements constitute a private, restricted-access network within the CHIN. When other projects are approved, such as the three described earlier in this chapter, access would be extended to include them as appropriate.

The Community Wellness Information Model

This project model uses a combination of a private network and the Internet to carry out its mission. The CHIN interaction with the public is over the Internet, while information sharing between the hospitals, the patient database, and the project is private. The

Figure 9.4 The Community Wellness Project Information Flow

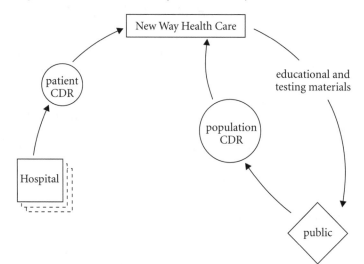

information flow in Figure 9.4 shows a CHIN that includes both the public network and the private network schematically. It also shows the two CDRs in two separate CISCs and the VSP.

This project has diverse information suppliers. New-Way Healthcare, on behalf of the community hospitals, supplies educational and testing materials. Each member of the community who uses the educational materials supplies information for evaluation and tracking project utilization. The hospitals supply extracted patient records for use in evaluation of the effectiveness of the wellness measures. The information users are the public and New-Way Healthcare.

Leveraging the Project

This project's assets are already being leveraged by extending its reach to include additional medical problems. Further leveraging might be done by taking advantage of the connectivity to the schools. For some of the project's medical problems, it might be appropriate to conduct clinical interventions such as immunizations or physical examinations at the schools. Clinical staff could add the results to the population database, as well as use the CHIN to update the students' records in the physicians' offices directly.

The population database itself contains enough demographic and health status information to be valuable for enterprise marketing and community planning for new healthcare resources. The CDR containing the extracted hospital records has a myriad of uses. Tying these and other multiuse aspects of the CHINs together is the subject of the next section.

INTEGRATING THE CHIN PROJECTS

CHIN initiators are almost always in the position of needing to generate support for a CHIN. These four projects show how broad a CHIN's support base can be, from health plans, hospitals, doctors, and consumers, to government agencies, schools, local business, and industry. An underplanned and undersold CHIN cannot get that support. The key factor to obtaining it is to show the specific and clear community value.

Each of the four CHIN projects described above has sufficient healthcare value to merit implementation as a stand-alone project. But there is no reason why a CHIN could not facilitate all these projects, even at the same time. Then, elements in each of the CHIN projects, and indeed even the projects themselves, become building blocks in a more mature CHIN. As noted before, the CHIN becomes more cost effective when its technology and infrastructure are fully utilized. It is especially cost effective when it serves multiple purposes.

The next several sections show the commonality of CHIN elements across all the projects, which becomes the motivating rationale for a CHIN.

Connectivity

Collectively these projects reach broadly into the community. The specific entities that are connected to the CHIN, and the reasons, are reviewed below.

Hospitals

Hospitals are connected so that they can contribute patient data for all four of the projects, but for a variety of reasons. Their contributions help to improve quality of care, monitor the incidence of specific medical problems, determine population health status, or market their services. They communicate primarily with the CDR or with one of the VSPs that is analyzing data. Hospitals also communicate through the CHIN with the health plans to access member information in the Enterprise Marketing Project.

Physicians

Physicians are connected to contribute patient data to the Quality Review and Mining Carryover Projects. They also access guidelines and educational materials in both of these projects. They communicate primarily with the VSP, and they can also access databases and educational materials over the Internet.

Consumers

Consumers are connected to access educational materials and games and to participate in evaluation and feedback over the Internet for the Community Wellness Project. Connectivity for them may be at home, at school, at a clinic, or even at the mall. Through the Internet, they access materials from the VSP and contribute to the population database.

Community groups

The Public Health Department, which is a government agency, and schools are two of the many non-healthcare delivery groups participating, for very different reasons. The government agency is actually conducting a project, the Mining Carryover Project, on the CHIN, while the schools are participating in the Community Wellness Project.

The Central Data Repositories

These projects collectively have defined two CDRs: a population data repository and a patient record data repository.

The patient record CDR

Information from patient records is used for every project, but entirely different slices of the record are used in each case. Because of the volume of inquiries, and for security purposes, it makes sense for a hospital to maintain a substantial extract of its enterprise patient database on the CHIN, rather than allowing repeated access to master records or repetitively supplying specific information on a case-by-case basis. Note again that the physical location of the records is immaterial. *Linkable access* is the key.

The population CDR

This data repository contains information about almost everyone in the community. It does not contain medical information, but it contains more health-related information than a medical record normally would. For example, it could contain such information as a record of exposure to environmental hazards or a record of wellness educational programs completed. A population database is needed in both the Mining Carryover and Community Wellness Projects. In the case of Mining Carryover, the VSP maintains its own population database. For the Community Wellness Project, the population database is part of the CHIN, but because it is connected to the Internet, it is kept and controlled in a separate CISC from the patient record database.

CHIN Information Service Centers

Each project has, or could have, a patient record CDR, and one has a population CDR as well, all of which are managed as a CISC of the CHIN. In addition, the CMPI is managed as its own CISC. Each of the first three projects uses the CMPI. The Quality Review Project uses it to acquire physician-specific information by linking a physician's patients' clinic and hospital records. The Enterprise Marketing Project uses it for plans that are affiliated with multiple hospitals, to link patient records across hospitals. The Mining Carryover Project uses it to link hospital and physician records to help detect environmentally-caused health problems. Although the Community Wellness Project uses two databases, they are not linked through the MPI because the patient database is used to monitor *populationwide* incidence of medical problems and is not tied to individual records in the population database.

Value-Added Service Providers

Even though all four projects require VSPs, these are the one type of CHIN element that is not redundant. Contracting with VSPs is a convenient way for a CHIN to obtain specialized services that are different for every project, especially in the early stages of the CHIN. However, it would be a mistake to consider VSPs as an entity apart from the CHIN. Since they often can be one of the central and most critical elements of a successful CHIN-based project, they are as much a CHIN participant as the information suppliers and the CISCs.

Brokering

Although brokering was explicitly discussed only in the Enterprise Marketing Project, it is a feature of every project. Interactions between every pair of elements in the CHIN are governed by brokering agreements. Although they are using the same transmission facilities and the same network management, the brokering agreements, including security measures, assure that only authorized correspondents can access or put information out over the CHIN. For instance, consumer access to the CHIN is only through the Internet, and only the population database receives data from the Internet.

Collaboration

Perhaps the most important common element in all these projects is the collaboration required to make them happen. It occurs at every level, from project conception, development, and oversight to gaining support, providing data, and participating in brokering. Sponsors collaborated in the Quality Review Project to launch the project and establish practice guidelines. They collaborated in the Enterprise Management Project to simplify a major reporting process for all healthcare enterprises. They collaborated in the Mining Carryover Project to acquire the data needed to protect the community's future. Finally, they collaborated in the Community Wellness Project to acquire the data needed to assess and improve community health.

CHINs work best when the healthcare infrastructure of a community takes responsibility for more than just caring for the sick in the same patterns as has been done throughout the tenure of "modern medicine." It's time for "post-modern medicine" to come to the fore. In each project, the CHIN enables the community healthcare system to go beyond—go outside the envelope—to reach out to new ways of fulfilling its mission.

Taking the first step toward collaboration is inevitably unnerving. One senses that, by unblocking the information flow, the business of community healthcare will never be the same. There are tough problems to be solved, such as deciding how to open up patient records for secondary purposes that benefit the community. Rather than serving as a reason not to collaborate, however, this issue should provide ample reason to begin the collaborative process. It is the only way the problem will be solved.

It is clear that genuine progress toward healthcare goals can be enabled by information flow in a way that never has been possible before. Once a collaborative relationship has been established, community stakeholders can begin to reap the benefits.

ELEMENTS OF THE UNIFYING CHIN

From a functional point of view, the three key CHIN responsibilities are managing the CISCs, proactively facilitating collaboration, and brokering. These are what distinguish a more sophisticated CHIN from a basic services information model. These are also what gives a CHIN its greatest value, by providing a means of sharing information (using the CISCs), sharing a collaborative framework, and sharing facilities (made possible by brokering). The four individual projects already show ample evidence of collaboration and brokering. What is needed now is to use the CHIN to integrate the four projects physically.

- The four patient record CDRs can be merged for the convenience of the hospitals, with the intention that the single CDR would be accessible by several projects.

- The two population databases, one managed by the CHIN and the other by a VSP, can be merged into one, managed by the CHIN and accessed by the VSP. This reduces project dependency on, and cost of, the Naples Services VSP from the Mining Carryover Project.

- The MPI, which heretofore was not linked to the population CDR, can be expanded to include the new population CDR. If it is also linked to CPRs in physicians' offices, it can be even more useful. At a minimum, it reduces project dependency on Biometrics Unlimited VSP in the Quality Review Project and on Naples Clinical Decision Support Services in the Mining Carryover Project.

- Physically, the projects are a collection of servers (e.g., VSPs, CISCs, hospitals, and plans) and workstations (e.g., office or school computers) connected to a telecommunications network. In many cases the servers (such as the CISCs and hospitals) and the workstations (such as the physicians' office computers) are the same for several projects. The CHIN is transparent in that the users of the servers and workstations cannot detect whether they are each operating on a separate CHIN or all on the same CHIN. The CHIN is responsible for the control of routing, access, and security that makes this possible.

THE UNIFYING CHIN

Figure 9.5 shows the Unifying CHIN with all the elements of the four projects combined or arranged on the network. Note particularly that part of the CHIN includes Internet access as a reminder that the CHIN is a concept that can have many physical representations.

THE NEXT ADDITIONS TO THE CHIN

The various project capabilities can be leveraged immediately in the Unifying CHIN. Here are several examples.

- Physician-to-physician and physician-to-patient electronic-mail capability could take advantage of the virtually community-wide connectivity. CHIN connectivity could further be used for electronic consultations. Office computer systems are available even now that are quite capable of providing videoconferencing capabilities, whereby two physicians can look at the same record at the same time and discuss it face-to-face via a video link. Ancillary diagnostic aids such as EKGs or x-rays, and even a look at or conversation with the patient, could also be shared via the video camera.

- Since mechanisms for community education programs are in place from the Community Wellness Project, educational material for the Mining Carryover Project could be added. Consumers could then begin to take responsibility themselves for recognizing health problems caused by Kaysburg's mining history.

Figure 9.5 The Unifying CHIN

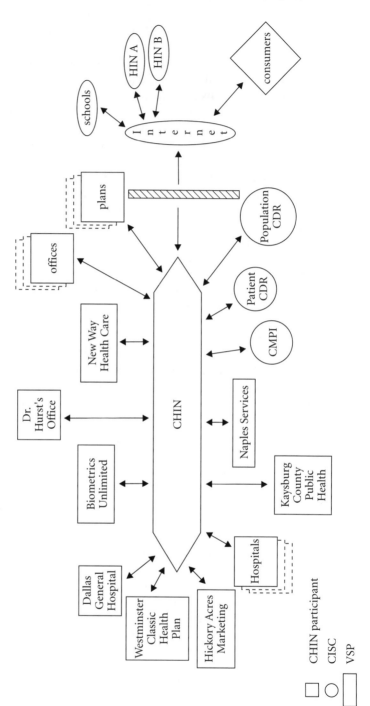

CHIN participant

CISC

VSP

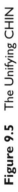

- Additional databases could easily be added to the CHIN. Possibilities include those suggested in Chapter 4, which contain information about community resources such as doctors, hospitals, other providers such as home health care agencies, and other community social resources.

- A financing system did not figure extensively in these projects because most healthcare executives are already familiar with how they might operate using a CHIN. Clearly, such a system would be an integral part of a Unifying CHIN.

- A VSP could generate the JCAHO and NCQA reports for hospitals and health plans.

- A VSP could manage complex projects in specific clinical areas over the Internet. For example, a VSP could design and implement a virtual conference or an interactive website.

- A VSP could manage customized continuing medical education programs for individual physicians, nurses, and other health professionals. It could select and deliver appropriate materials over the CHIN and then evaluate and register credits.

- Much of what a VSP would do now will be routine CHIN functions in the future. For example, when all community providers participate in maintaining the patient record CDR, then the VSP function of data acquisition from multiple clinical sources for analysis will no longer be necessary. Also, clinical guidelines for virtually all conditions will have been developed, so the task becomes one of maintenance and updating. Instead of replacing VSPs, however, the VSPs would make even more specialized and sophisticated contributions, enabled by such expanded CHIN tools as greater connectivity and the availability of essential databases.

- Although the extracted patient record CDR is actually intended only for post-clinical care use such as research, many of the concepts embedded in it, such as sharing information and establishment of data standards and medical terminology standards, are applicable to development of a communitywide CPR. The much-discussed continuum of care, whereby a person has a single lifetime medical record, will only be possible when communities begin to work toward such a CPR.

COMMUNITY HEALTH INFORMATION SYSTEMS

The Unifying CHIN described here clearly is more inclusive than most CHINs today. Yet it is no more sophisticated technically, nor does it require any more networking resources, than today's CHINs. The difference is in the collaborative approach to solving community health care problems rather than providing administrative simplification for community enterprises. When a CHIN has matured to the point of being truly integrated into the community healthcare infrastructure as an indispensable resource and fully committed partner in meeting the goals of the healthcare system, it might more properly be called a CHIS—a Community Health Information System.

CHAPTER 10

BEYOND THE CHIN

The scenarios thus far have treated the CHIN in relative isolation, relying almost exclusively on community resources (the exception being the Internet). Even community healthcare enterprises for the most part played the passive role of allowing data use. This approach, while probably unrealistic, allowed the examples to highlight fresh aspects of CHINs. As it matures into a system, or CHIS, however, a CHIN increasingly will interact with, affect, and be affected by its environment

When the CHIN does begin to interact fully with its participant enterprises and with the healthcare system beyond its community boundaries, the synergy is awesome to contemplate. This chapter explores the issues and potential at these two interfaces. CHIN interaction with participant enterprises focuses on the CPR, which clearly is at the heart of all clinical uses of the CHIN. Its interaction with the rest of the healthcare system is assessed by review of developments in progress nationwide. It shows how these elements converge to achieve a national health information system. Such a system brings added resources and capabilities to the CHIN and heightens its impact and value within the community even further.

THE COMPUTER-BASED PATIENT RECORD

The single most important relationship between enterprise and CHIN is sharing the CPR. From the earliest days of information systems in the 1960s, medical informaticians have envisioned a patient record that was readily available when and where needed, complete and accurate, and that could be integrated with clinical advice whenever the record was opened. Such a record could only be achieved with information technology, and as the technology matured over the next 30 years, so did the vision. Implementation of the vision, however, has scarcely progressed beyond the experimental. Since the CPR is essential to CHIN vitality, it is important to understand just where healthcare enterprises stand with respect to its implementation.

Historical Perspective on CPR Concepts

CPR concepts are as old as the information technology that has enabled storing patient information, merging the record with clinical advice, and making it available in multiple locations. Consider the following historical progression of CPR concepts as they relate to CHINs.

- The record was never perceived as an end in itself, but was originally conceived of as a tool for optimal management of a patient's care.

- As information technology became more powerful, it became clear that this same patient record would also be the best source for all the management, accounting, and financial information needed by the provider, rather than maintaining separate administrative systems.

- When quality assessment became the norm, again it was clear that the tasks of quality assurance or utilization review, for instance, could only be performed adequately by a computer system that could assess care by examining CPRs.

- When reminder systems (such as those that advise a doctor of a patient's drug allergies or drug interactions when placing a drug order in the record) and care paths became popular, it was clear that guidelines on the large scale needed for complete patient care could be incorporated into the patient record only if the record were computer based.

- More recently, the countless unanswered questions in healthcare have fueled the notion that patient records might actually be a viable source of raw data for clinical and health services research. For the first time, the idea took hold that patient information in general might have value beyond that of the care of the patient. If patient records were fully automated and available, the billions of heretofore wasted bits of information might serve multiple secondary purposes.

- Even though the medical portions of patient records have not been tapped through a CPR for research, substantial portions of the records began to be captured by providers and plans for marketing and quality analyses.

- The realization today is that, given access to CPRs through a CHIN, the secondary uses of clinical information could go beyond the aforementioned research, marketing, and quality assessment for institutions. The information could also be used by VSPs to develop educational materials, guidelines, and resource management, and by community agencies to set and carry out healthcare policy.

- Since the CPR would be available through the CHIN, a patient record would no longer necessarily be tied to the provider that generated it. It could become the record of the continuum of care, containing all relevant information about the patient from all providers and even from the patient and his or her environment.

- Since all providers could have access to the CPR over the CHIN, electronic clinical collaboration using e-mail or videoconferencing could replace the traditional but temporally unsatisfactory clinical consultation.

CPR Concepts vs. Reality

As CPR concepts have matured to keep pace with new information technology, so have ideas about the range of impact of the CPR. The CPR was envisioned to evolve as a unifying and foundational concept in these progressively expanding locales:

- a specialty service or clinic;
- an entire hospital or clinic;
- a healthcare delivery enterprise with several institutional components;
- a community, shared among several healthcare delivery enterprises;
- a community, including non-healthcare delivery enterprises; and
- a regional, state, or national resource with multiple purposes.

Although all these various concepts of the role of patient information are the subject of research and implementation, not one of them, including even the most basic concept of using the CPR as a patient management tool, has achieved wide-spread acceptance as an essential element of the healthcare process or of the healthcare system. Yet clearly, the CPR is integral to the continuing maturation of healthcare and evolution toward society's goals.

At the same time as CPR concepts were maturing and research intensifying, information technology also increasingly supported automation of the patient record for nonclinical purposes. However, actual use of the CPR has followed quite a different progression from the one envisioned. Instead it has followed this very limited path:

- institutional care of individual patients;
- institutional claims processing;
- institutional proof of quality of care;
- intraenterprise administration of patient care; and
- enterprise marketing.

Other envisioned uses of patient information such as the quality assurance equation are not yet priority items at the enterprise or national level. However, a CPR is essential to most CHIN goals, so healthcare executives must be aware of the role of the CPR and then create the conditions under which it can be achieved, first at the enterprise level and then at the community level. Table 10.1 summarizes that role, from its short-term use in patient care to its secondary use within the enterprise, the community, and beyond.

The CHIN should facilitate development of enterprise CPRs. Consider the CHIN infrastructure as a tool that makes the task easier to do than each enterprise could do alone. The collaborative nature of the CHIN makes it possible on a community basis to develop or adapt

Table 10.1 The Role of the Computer-Based Patient Record Over Time

	Locus of Use	Purposes
Immediate	Encounter site	Patient care
Short term	Enterprise	Management Planning Quality assessment Accreditation
Midterm	Community	Continuum of care Consultation Collaboration Quality assurance Public health monitoring Wellness planning
Long term	Healthcare system	Medical knowledge base Guidelines Research Education Policy

standards, build prototypes, and conduct pilot studies together. The results benefit all community enterprises and level the playing field for competition on parameters that really matter to the community.

The CPR's strategic, as well as practical, value to the enterprise cannot be overestimated. Increasingly, healthcare enterprises will be judged by the extent of their contributions to the community, and by evidence of their leadership in solving the problems of the troubled healthcare system, rather than by how privately they can hold themselves. The fully evolved healthcare system awaits enterprises who act in the best interests of the system. Healthcare executives must understand that enterprise CPRs, developed according to agreed-upon national standards, are the ticket to personal and enterprise credibility in the quality-driven healthcare system of the future.

NATIONAL SUPPORT FOR THE CPR

Enterprises that decide to develop a CPR either in house or in collaboration with other CHIN enterprises are not alone. Since several medical centers have developed and used CPRs successfully for years, good models are available. Among these are The Medical Record at Duke University Medical Center, the Regenstrief Medical Record System at Indiana University Medical Center, the Harvard Community Health Plan system, the Department of Veterans Affairs model, and the Department of Defense model.

A major national study conducted by the Institute of Medicine concluded CPRs were essential for coping with the increasingly complex information management requirements of healthcare (Dick and Steen 1991). The study recommended joint public and private sector establishment of "a Computer-Based Patient Record Institute (CPRI) to promote and facilitate development, implementation, and dissemination of the CPR."

The Washington-based CRPI was indeed established. It functions according to the blueprint laid out by the Institute of Medicine study, facilitating standards development activities by several groups; offering educational programs; studying critical CPR issues such as confidentiality, security, infrastructure, legislation, and archiving; and promoting demonstration projects.

CHIN-TO-CHIN COLLABORATION

Mature CHINs of the future, or CHISs, will routinely collaborate on programs for which a larger population or a greater concentration of professional expertise would create additional value. Such collaboration could be regional, for instance, when several CHINs in the same state might pool resources, contracting with a VSP to meet common

Figure 10.1   A Regional Health Information System

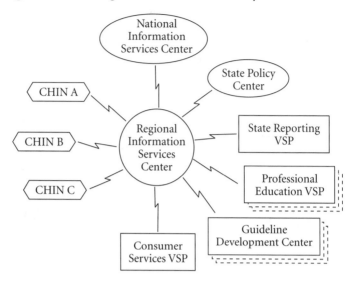

state reporting requirements, develop educational materials, or produce guidelines. Figure 10.1 shows the resulting linkage schematically as a Regional Health Information System (RHIS). When needs are common to every community in the country, such as the need for the latest research information, the collaboration could extend even further to create a NHIS, shown schematically in Figure 10.2 (Duncan 1994). Here are several examples already discussed as CHIN capabilities that extend CHIN capabilities to systems on a larger scale.

The Medical Knowledge Base

The dynamic medical knowledge base is a national resource, parts of which reside all over the country at every medical center, school, and library. Information technology has already proven to be the key to ready access, since much of the medical literature is available over the Internet or by connecting directly to the National Library of Medicine (NLM) through Medline. It is available because community enterprises, government agencies, and publishers choose to share their resources nationally, using information technology.

Development of Guidelines

Guideline development is an excellent example of how every community can contribute its patient data and professional expertise to improving health services for all communities. Although examples

Figure 10.2 The National Health Information System

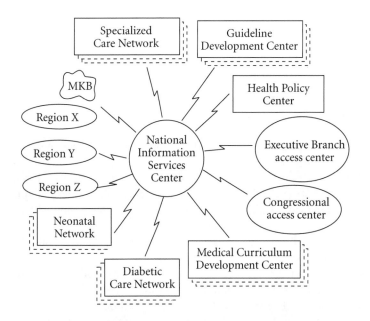

throughout the book have shown guideline development at the community level, it is not always appropriate or necessary. Rare medical conditions may not be recognized by many community physicians. Complex medical conditions often require more attention than community physicians are able to devote to studying them. In such cases, a single community probably does not have the resources, including the time to research and study, to develop more than a few of the more complex guidelines. With CHIN-to-CHIN linkages, the work can be shared among a national pool of experts on every subject.

Consider the possibility of national VSPs, called guideline development centers, each of which has the ability to tap national expertise in a particular area of clinical medicine. The centers would be based at medical centers throughout the country. For example, consider a center with expertise in blood vessel disease that is developing guidelines for use of carotid endarterectomy. Connecting to CHINs through the NHIS, the center would 1) collect data from CDRs, or directly from CPRs, on patients with blood vessel disease, 2) tap the MKB for all relevant research findings, 3) perhaps commission additional research studies, and 4) provide facilities for electronic collaboration of experts. The experts would work collaboratively over the NHIS to study the background materials, deliberate, and then develop the content of the guidelines.

The guidelines, which would be kept updated by the same center, would be available for use by community physicians throughout the country, and they could be modified for local use as practical. For example, a community that has a high incidence of skin diseases might expand a national guideline in that area to include more detail.

Quality Medical Education

Each medical school has its own curriculum and its own style of medical record keeping, and its faculty have varying levels and types of expertise. It is not surprising that medical practice shows so much variation from community to community and even hospital to hospital. This variability highlights the dangers of community-based—or even worse, enterprise-based—standards of care. From the point of view of the consumer, at least, curriculum and standards for use in medical education, including record keeping, should be set nationally, as part of the quality of care improvement process.

VSPs called medical curriculum development centers could be created to work analogously to the guideline development centers to develop and maintain specific pieces of the medical school curriculum. Clearly, their work would rely heavily on the clinical guidelines developed by their sister centers, so medical school graduates would leave school ready to use the guidelines—and the CPR. In previous examples the CHIN was used to deliver educational materials to community physicians and consumers. With the current example, it is possible for the NHIS, including the CHINs, to deliver entire curricula electronically.

Wellness and Public Health

The CHIN has been shown to serve public health by providing the means to correlate community medical problems with environmental factors. The CHIN or a larger system could as well serve national public health by correlating patient behavior and population information with not only environmental factors but also factors from other social systems such as education or welfare. A critical first step is to access community information from CDRs, CPRs, or both through the many CHINs.

NEW CAPABILITIES

Clinical medicine can look for help in many new ways when the NHIS, including CHISs and RHISs, is in place. Healthcare executives may be intrigued by many of these examples.

Disease Management

The relatively new mode of healthcare delivery called disease management offers fresh challenges to healthcare information management.

Since interventions are out of the hands of traditional providers and may occur at several locations throughout a community, management of the record keeping aspects alone would justify a CHIN in areas where use of disease management is widespread.

The concept of disease management makes good sense for the healthcare system, since it distributes patient care to ancillary providers who relieve primary providers of repetitive care such as home visits, patient education, and monitoring for compliance with doctor's instructions. However, well-grounded research is lacking to fully support disease management. The NHIS has a role to play in facilitating such research and establishing national standards for the benefit of all communities.

Specialty Care Networks

Outpatient specialty care centers are ubiquitous for well-defined purposes such as kidney dialysis or management of diabetes. Because the orientation is on care delivery, there is a risk that our understanding of the disease processes and therapies may stagnate. The NHIS can offer a way to vitalize such centers. For example, the MidPeninsula Diabetic Care Center, a hypothetical organization, is a part of such a network, the Diabetic Care Network. Here is what the Network does for them:

- National Diabetic Care, a VSP, maintains a resource database of all centers, physicians, and directories relating to diabetes.
- It maintains a customized search program to all the literature on diabetes.
- A weekly bulletin of new research findings and resources relating to diabetes is sent over the network to MidPeninsula.
- National Diabetic Care develops and distributes standards for CPRs, designed especially to meet diabetic care centers' needs.
- The common CPR standards make it possible for research teams to use the facilities of the network and National Diabetic Care (or another research-oriented VSP) to routinely conduct clinical research related to diabetes and health services research aimed at advancing diabetic care delivery.
- The VSP prepares educational materials, which can be distributed to patients in paper form, video form, or over the network.
- Patients can use e-mail to communicate with the center for appointments or with questions about their problems or their care.

High-Risk Networks

Fast-breaking developments characterize some areas of medicine such as the care of high-risk newborns. Saint George Medical Center, which supports a sophisticated center for neonatal care, participates in the national Neonatal Network. The central capability of that network is its capacity for collaborative clinical research and consultation. New research findings, or even ideas, are disseminated immediately via the network for real-time discussion and feedback. Saint George's physicians particularly like the weekly neonatal "Rounds," during which participating centers present their babies with particularly challenging or educational problems to a national audience over the network. Other services provided are similar to those available over the Diabetic Care Network for physician and patient support.

Support for Rare or Complex Disorders

Extensive anecdotal evidence describes patients whose medical problems were not diagnosed or treated in their own communities. Their national searches for someone who could help them are often heartbreaking. The Internet already has put a wealth of medical information and resources at their fingertips, but with the help of the healthcare system, much more could be done for such people, as the following examples illustrate:

- Physicians should have available resource directories of physicians and facilities, organized in several useful dimensions such as chief complaint or disease category. They should be able to contact these resources directly on behalf of their patients— in other words, a national electronic consultation. With this support, the community physician may be able to retain and care for the patient.

- Electronic decision support systems based on disease or even patient models would help physicians to discriminate between what is known and what is new. For patients with recognizable problems, such systems would also be able to generate individually based guidelines, specific for the patient. For problems not previously encountered, the systems would continuously refine the medical knowledge base as they come to "know" each puzzling new patient, thus pointing to new directions for clinical research.

- Electronic-mail support groups should be much more widely available for patient-to-patient communication, as part of a move toward encouraging self-care.

Complex Levels of Research

Healthcare does not always lend itself to an orderly examination of things such as cause and effect relationships on an individual level. Consider these three examples:

- Although many risk factors are known for heart disease on a population basis, little is known as to why many individuals do not follow the pattern. Some people at high risk do not develop heart disease, while others with no risk factors do.
- Genetic research depends on our ability to link records across generations. Family trees indicating the presence or absence of a disease or a gene are inadequate; entire records are needed for study.
- The impact of prenatal nutrition and care on the health and development of babies may be much greater than physicians imagine, with wide-ranging social implications. Research in this area would require the ability to link a comprehensive maternal record with a comprehensive record of the baby's health and development.

Research on these kinds of problems requires an information infrastructure for healthcare beyond our most visionary hopes for the CPR. Once a standardized CPR is routinely in use throughout the healthcare system, designers can turn their attention to conceptualizing and realizing these more sophisticated systems.

Changing the Locus of Care

A full set of clinical decision support tools, including guidelines for care, CPRs throughout the system, a fully realized and accessible MKB, and ubiquitous computer workstations, combine to deliver the capability to examine and treat patients in diverse locations. Several examples used in this book include storefront clinics, homes, schools, institutions, and the workplace. With such extensive support, new types of providers whose training is targeted to use the tools could deliver lower-cost care at these locations. Patients would need to go to the traditional centralized clinics only for specialized care.

THE HEALTHCARE INFRASTRUCTURE

A solid healthcare infrastructure might be able to break the vicious escalation of compensatory dissonance, described in Chapter 2, that dominates the system today. Both internal management of the healthcare system and informed policy formation affecting healthcare are needed.

Internal Management

Although the body of medical knowledge is vast, it is substantially, and to some extent unnecessarily, incomplete. Further, our ability to bring that knowledge to bear on patients' current or potential problems in an orderly and convincing way has not kept pace with the development of new medical knowledge. As a result of this and other factors, the quality of the healthcare system itself—even beyond quality of care—is rising rapidly to the top of the list of important health system issues.

With the connectivity of an NHIS, the healthcare system could begin to take responsibility for implementing the quality assurance cycle on a national scale. It could begin to assess its resources and plan for those needed, such as physicians, hospitals, or centers of excellence in specific clinical arenas. It would be able to establish national standards for medical education. It would be able to conduct health services research routinely on the organization and financing of healthcare. It would be able to implement subnetworks such as the Diabetic Care Network or a Guideline Development Network as national resources. In short, if the healthcare system had structure, leadership, and HINs, it would have the tools to manage itself.

National Policy

Legislators throughout the political spectrum believe that HINs are central to our ability to improve healthcare quality and access while lowering costs. Within an NHIS, legislators and regulators would be able to create policy subsystems analogous to the quality and education subsystems described earlier. They could use these subsystems to direct research and obtain the information and analyses they need for informed and intelligent, rather than ad hoc, policy formation for healthcare.

SUMMARY

A critical mass of healthcare stakeholders needs access to community, regional, and national networks before information technology can begin to meet the needs of the healthcare system as a whole. As discussed in Chapter 4, these needs revolve around breaking the information logjam in healthcare. The above examples have shown some of the possibilities that would open up for policy, quality assurance, education, patient care, clinical research, and access to the MKB. Without information technology, none of these would be possible.

Prospects for a National Health Information System

Momentum toward an NHIS was observed as long ago as the late 1970s (Duncan 1980). In recent years the idea has gained momentum as part of the White House's High Performance Computing and

Communications (HPCC) program, which is developing the enabling technologies on which a National Information Infrastructure can be built (High Performance Computing and Communications Program 1997). Although the HPCC program is being developed with federal money, it is anticipated that it will be built and operated by the private sector.

The NII would be a national network much like the Internet in concept, except that it would address societal needs (Lindberg and Humphreys 1995). Every citizen would have access. A NHIS would operate as a subsystem on such a network, along with networks (using the same communications capabilities) for other social areas such as education, energy management, and the environment. Key government healthcare players are the National Library of Medicine (NLM) and the Agency for Health Care Policy and Research (AHCPR). Even with federal support for the information infrastructure, many nontechnology issues still need to be resolved.

Because the need for information flow in healthcare is so great, it is likely that an NHIS will eventually be mandated, if only so that the government can fulfill its oversight role. Instead of this top-down approach to achieving the NHIS, healthcare executives for community enterprises and other leaders in the healthcare system may prefer to create the system themselves, bottom-up, beginning with CHINs.

References · · · · · · · · · · · · ·

Dick, R. S., and E. B. Steen (eds.). *The Computer-Based Patient Record: An Essential Technology for Health Care*. Washington, DC: National Academy Press.

Duncan, K. A. (1980). "The Trend Toward a National Health Information System in the United States." In *Proceedings of Medinfo '80*, edited by D. A. B. Lindberg and S. Kaihara. 663–68. Amsterdam: North-Holland.

Duncan, K. A. 1994. *Health Information and Health Reform: Understanding the Need for a National Health Information System*. San Francisco: Jossey-Bass.

"High Performance Computing and Communications Program FY 1997 Implementation Plan." http://www.hppc.gov/imp97/.

Lindberg, D. A. B., and B. L. Humphreys. 1995. "The High-Performance Computing and Communications Program, the National Information Infrastructure, and Health Care." *Journal of the American Medical Informatics Association* 2 (3):156–59.

CHAPTER 11

PROSPECTS AND RECOMMENDATIONS FOR ACHIEVING CHINS

The healthcare system needs CHINs that can mature into full
CHIS and break the healthcare information logjam. Barriers
to this achievement cascade through the system at every level—
offices, enterprises, communities, the system itself, and society. These
barriers are not discrete; rather, they are interdependent, each affecting others. This chapter discusses the barriers to meaningful
progress, beginning with technology and societal factors and pro-
gressing through the system to CHINs, enterprises, and offices. An
example of the cycle of interdependence of many barriers highlights the need to break the cycle. The chapter and book conclude
with recommendations to national organizations to take the lead
in creating a climate where CHINs can flourish, and to healthcare executives to shape a healthier future for their enterprises and
communities.

TECHNOLOGY-BASED BARRIERS

The barriers to health information networks are no longer technology
based. The computing power, the data storage capacity, the transmission speed, and the cryptography to provide confidentiality, while not
fully mature, are sufficiently well developed to enable communities
to generate highly useful healthcare information systems, including
CHINs.

Healthcare executives are perhaps too well aware that, despite the sophistication of essential information technology tools, new technologies and approaches are emerging faster than ever. Virtual reality, artificial intelligence, graphic interfaces, new input devices, videoconferencing, and telemedicine all show great promise. We are told that the Internet is in its infancy and that no one can accurately imagine the capabilities it will offer in just a few years. It seems natural to question the value of today's initiatives when better ones could be taken tomorrow.

Thus the technology today becomes a barrier when it overpowers those who want to use it, creating a self-defeating paralysis of will. Enterprises in particular cling to their legacy systems because the strength of their vision of the information-rich future does not match their uncertainty about technology directions.

SOCIETAL BARRIERS

Agreement is widespread, even in Congress, that the healthcare system needs information technology to carry out its business. Yet the national will to achieve the required systems is lacking. The responsibility lies in large part with those who understand and advocate the complex vision of healthcare in an information society, yet have failed to translate it in a way that will capture the national imagination.

Another prime barrier lies in the deeply clinical aspects of healthcare information technology. The traditional respect with which policymakers have always viewed clinicians has heretofore prevented them from mandating the use of such a powerful clinical agent as HINs would surely be. This barrier will fall in the short term to the perception of need for oversight of managed care organizations and, longer term, to the need to restore the eroding infrastructure of healthcare (access, education, and research).

The privacy issue is yet another barrier. It is a poorly understood issue, in terms both of the nature of the threat and the remedies available. It is also a paradoxical issue. On the one hand, many who might support HINs are afraid to do so because of the privacy issue. On the other hand, this country has never had a privacy crisis of sufficient magnitude to trigger a national insistence on measures to ensure confidentiality.

SYSTEMWIDE BARRIERS

The flawed healthcare system, which lacks goal-directed leadership and an infrastructure within which to plan and manage its affairs, is itself a barrier to HINs. The very words, *network* and *system*, connote collaboration and synergism. The healthcare system needs to work proactively to end the traditional information isolation of its large and small competitive cottage industries. As long as it does not do so, the system remains a barrier.

BARRIERS IN MEDICAL INFORMATICS

Medical informaticians have been working for decades on the tough problems faced by those who want to use information technology in healthcare. A great contribution of the discipline has been the accessibility of the published medical literature via Medline. Progress on data standards and medical vocabularies for the CPR are also due to medical informatics initiatives. On the whole, however, the discipline is insular and short-sighted. Too many of its scientists work at the level of the laboratory bench rather than at the level of the system. While such work must be done, the emphasis must be shifted to include systems issues, in order to bring the healthcare system out of crisis. As an example, consider that the discipline's work toward standards and medical vocabularies may soon lead to an ideally designed CPR. The problem is, who in the healthcare system would be prepared to use it? Each medical school in the country teaches a different system of record keeping. Even if the process of change in the schools begins soon, it may take decades to bring every physician into using the ideal CPR. Thus, medical informaticians should extend their mission beyond *developing* the CPR to *integrating* it into common use in the healthcare system.

CHIN BARRIERS

Current conceptions of CHINs center on information technology–based capabilities such as data transmission and access to databases such as laboratory test results or claims status. Moving to the next level beyond these basic capabilities will undoubtedly involve creating an MPI and a CDR for secondary use of at least part of a CPR. These in turn raise the issues of a standard medical vocabulary, standards for data representation and transmission, assurance of data quality, confidentiality of information, and ownership of data. Since these issues affect every community healthcare enterprise, it only makes sense that the solutions lie in collaborative action.

Even when these issues are resolved at the community level, more needs to be done to achieve a CHIS. Most of the scenarios in this book stress that the value of the CHIN lies in its goal-directed, value-added use. The greatest barrier to achieving that value is a reluctance by enterprises to collaborate on goal-directed programs such as the quality feedback cycle, the wellness and environmental monitoring programs, or the inner-city access project.

The second barrier might be observed to be a failure of imagination. Healthcare executives and other community leaders experience daily the gap between healthcare needs and the partial solutions being delivered. Too many CHINs start with an empty shell of connectivity, without the accompanying effort to create value. Schools, government agencies, businesses, and civic organizations need first to pool their creativity to understand the community's health status, to assess its needs, and to set goals. They then need to pool their resources to achieve those goals. It sounds simple, but it's not happening.

ENTERPRISE BARRIERS

The uncertainty with which many, if not most, healthcare enterprises live has been cited often. Their efforts to reduce their costs have many untoward consequences that have become barriers to health information networks. The focus on cost cutting dilutes the focus on the healthcare system goals that should be the goals of the CHIN. That focus has also led to a reduction in the education and research missions of many institutions, which in time will translate into a weakening of the healthcare infrastructure. The need in some enterprises for shareholder profit maintains the price purchasers pay for healthcare, rather than reducing the price. At the same time it is removing billions of dollars from the healthcare system that could have been used to address the quality and access problems. Too many enterprises that are not-for-profit are largely struggling to survive. In short, the enterprise environment in general is not conducive to the community outreach required for CHINs.

The discussion of CHIN dependency on enterprises, for patient data, and for collaboration to resolve the attendant issues places the ability of the CHIN to mature squarely in the hands of the enterprises. Healthcare executives understand that each enterprise must develop a CPR. Many simply do not think they can afford to do so, or do not see an approach that makes sense for them. They should know, however, that the longer they cling to their legacy systems, the more work it will take to move ahead later. Equally problematic are the many large enterprises that are developing their own systems. At best these systems are of unknown compatibility with the rest of healthcare.

INTERDEPENDENCY OF BARRIERS

Almost all barriers in turn have their own barriers to solution. For example, hospitals, clinics, and individual doctors are urged to adopt a CPR, not just to share information through a CHIN, but primarily because a CPR means better patient care. They most likely would plan to acquire such a system from a vendor rather than to develop their own. Vendors need to offer standards-driven CPRs, but compliance with standards is an ill-defined process for which vendors probably would argue that they lack sufficient guidance (Hammond 1997). Moreover, the economics of offering a CPR are defeating when one considers that every doctor and hospital must have a slightly different one. A standard CPR probably cannot be realized until a standard medical record is realized. Presumably, if anyone truly knew what should be put in a medical record, and where and why, and for how long, and if they could predict its relevance in every case, then such a record could be conceived (Weed 1993). This in turn awaits a more complete medical knowledge base.

RECOMMENDATIONS

Specific and detailed recommendations for developing CHINs have been made by Wakerly and by Benton International (Benton International 1994). The informational, technical, and project management processes are complex, with many new facets, but they are also straightforward. The recommendations in this book go beyond those processes to emphasize the need to change the environment for CHINs.

This chapter's recommendations, then, for the healthcare system, policymakers, and medical informaticians concentrate first on creating a climate conducive to creativity and growth for CHINs. Subsequent to these recommendations are more specific proposals for action by enterprises and CHINs. Final recommendations are for healthcare executives who are guiding enterprises toward their information-rich vision of a goal-focused healthcare system.

The National Environment for CHINs

In a healthcare system that seems devoid of the focus and leadership essential for solving its problems, concerned national groups must begin to fill the need for direction and advocacy. Examples of several of the kinds of groups that can and should act are listed here:

Department of Health and Human Services Public Health Service
- National Library of Medicine
- Agency for Health Care Policy and Research

Healthcare Organizations
- American Medical Association
- American Hospital Association
- American College of Physicians

- American Nursing Association
- American Healthcare Information Management Association
- Association for Health Services Research
- American Public Health Association
- American College of Healthcare Executives
- Association of American Medical Colleges

Accrediting and Evaluating Groups

- Joint Commission on Accreditation of Healthcare Organizations
- National Committee for Quality Assurance
- Health Care Financing Administration

Medical Informatics Groups

- American Medical Informatics Association
- Computer-Based Patient Records Institute
- Health Level Seven
- Healthcare Information and Management Systems Society

Specific recommendations call for such national groups to become proactive advocates and facilitators in several key areas.

Ending information isolation

On behalf of the healthcare system and the society it serves, healthcare institutions such as professional societies, accrediting bodies, and related government agencies need to work to end the culture of information isolation that pervades the system. Although fears about confidentiality are legitimate and must be allayed, the issue has for too long served as a reason for systemic inaction. The tasks to be accomplished are arduous and expensive in the short term, but delay only makes them more so. Moreover, the payoff in terms of health and healthcare is many times more valuable than the cost. Besides the need to continue developing the CPR, two primary aspects of information isolation need to be addressed at the national level.

1. We continue to graduate a population of doctors who have not studied adequately the nature and role of information in healthcare and how to use it. Furthermore, these new doctors' practices collectively will use hundreds of different methods of record keeping. National organizations must supply the rationale and motivation for the curriculum changes that need to be defined and implemented.

2. New enterprise information systems are being added daily. Each new system adds to the burden of legacy systems that eventually must be integrated, one by one, into CHINs. To achieve

compatibility from the outset, national organizations need to generate the rationale and motivation for enterprise and CHIN adoption of standards at every level, from medical vocabulary to data definitions to communications.

Implementing the quality assurance equation

A CHIN that focuses on improving the quality of care relies heavily on national resources, especially for access to the electronically available medical literature. But this access is limited in its usefulness for improving quality. Guideline developers have learned that the published literature alone is not very useful to community physicians. The MKB needs to present an organized body of knowledge to physicians and others, with new research findings from the literature incorporated as appropriate. Studies are being commissioned to fill in the gaps in the dynamic MKB, but even these are not enough. New styles of routine and ongoing clinical research are needed. The MKB must "know" how to access, analyze, and incorporate the vast untapped database of patient information in CPRs throughout the country. While full use of information in CPRs may be decades away, national organizations need to start now to lay the conceptual groundwork for achieving such an MKB.

Creating subsystems

The vision of an NHIS may never be achieved if its development continues to progress on an institution-by-institution basis. Current demonstration projects focus too narrowly on institutional use in isolation, whereas real impact on health and healthcare needs a national push. Ideas can be leveraged by providing communities with incentives to create CHINs. Positive national incentives would come from programs such as those suggested in the next paragraph.

National organizations, especially professional societies and government agencies, need to begin implementing nationally networked subsystems appropriate for their areas of expertise. The objective should go further than simply making information available, as is the case with most websites today. Rather, the objective should be to make a measurable difference in health and healthcare. For example, an oncology-focused professional society or foundation could commit to creating a high-risk network like that described in Chapter 10. Associations and foundations concerned about medical education could collaborate to gain support for medical school curriculum and pedagogy reform and then work toward its implementation. The key is to work toward systemwide change that will both encourage development of health information networks and then use them to best advantage.

The Role of Medical Informatics

The business of medical informatics is serving healthcare. Leaders of this multidisciplinary field need to create an information model, based on healthcare system goals, that goes beyond the process of clinical care to encompass all factors relating to health and healthcare, including consideration of the system's environment. The discipline should then make certain its research agendas and educational programs focus on the toughest of the barriers to realization of the model. Agenda items would surely go beyond development of infrastructure and tools to include developing models for collaboration at all levels, including innovative models for clinical research and education; solving the problems of knowledge representation in the MKB; creating interfaces that make the MKB relevant and useful to medical education, clinical practice, and individuals; and study and resolution of societal, sociological, and psychological issues related to the optimal adoption of the technology.

Recommendations for CHIN Activists

CHIN initiators and directors need most to be more imaginative and aggressive and to avoid underpromising what the CHIN can deliver. Thinking with folded hands needs to give way to assessing proactively the community's potential for good health and quality healthcare and then creating the information models that will become the basis for mature CHINs. Who does not have access to care? Where are the health threats? What medical problems are not well managed? Is there a better way to organize care? Think in terms of collaborative solutions and value-added services, reaching into all corners, including schools, businesses, community groups, and government agencies.

CHIN initiators and directors also need to look beyond the healthcare enterprises for support, stressing the CHIN's ability to leverage assets throughout the community. Moving results from laboratories to offices and processing claims have both been accomplished without a computer for many years, and they do not inspire participation from the community at large. Many communities may have groups such as Joint Venture: Silicon Valley in Northern California, which is a public-private coalition dedicated to the revitalization of the Valley. One of its projects is Smart Valley, which facilitates information technology networks for education, healthcare, and public access to government. Such a group, or even a chamber of commerce, should serve as a rallying point for support from the community.

Recommendations for Enterprises

A recurring theme in this book is for enterprises to focus on community needs and goals for healthcare and to collaborate in meeting those goals. Collaboration should take many forms, not the least of which is working with community and other partners to:

- adopt standards;
- devise a CMPI;
- renew their commitment to implementing an enterprise CPR;
- agree on the contents of one or more CDRs based on their CPRs; and
- implement security measures ranging from protection of confidentiality to network reliability to recovery from natural disasters.

Standards collaboration should build on the work of national standards organizations. Early emphasis needs to be given to a CMPI that (1) uniquely identifies a patient through a biometric identification, (2) contains sufficient basic identifying information, conforming to standards, to match records at different locations, and (3) uses a reliable method of finding and linking records. Security measures must be end-to-end, encompassing not only information while it is on the CHIN, but also within the enterprise.

Within the enterprise, working toward higher data quality is paramount. Even within the hospital or clinic, information may be viewed and used many times. Its potential for secondary use is limitless, as shown in Table 10.1, and high-quality data may command a high price. Patient records are indeed an untapped information resource for research, policy formation, education, and support of quality improvement, but the guarantee of data quality must be unquestionable.

Professional and administrative staff throughout the enterprise need to share in the mission and goals for healthcare, but they also need to think of their own roles with more flexibility and creativity. In addition to caring for people when they are ill, they need to feel accountable to the community as a whole by taking whatever responsibility they can for keeping people healthy. Constructing and sharing an accurate and complete patient record is part of this commitment. Enterprise programs that include training, incentives, and monitoring are needed to achieve consistently high data quality.

Recommendations for Healthcare Executives

It must be clear to healthcare executives who have read this book that the enterprises they manage are critical to the CHIN effort. Their cooperation in goal setting and collaboration to create the informational and technical infrastructure is essential. It is the vision and commitment of the healthcare executives that will make it happen.

As a practical matter, healthcare executives need to take both a short and a long view of CHINs. The only viable short-term approach to launching CHINs may well be to obtain commitments from key enterprises to use a CHIN for administrative simplification and cost savings, with some access to clinical applications, including telemedicine.

In the long term, however, the arguments for goal-directed CHINs are unassailable, benefiting the enterprises as much or more than any other stakeholder except the consumers of healthcare. Rather than dwelling on the difficulties, healthcare executives are urged to seek areas where there is agreement and begin constructing the building blocks that will lead to mature CHINs, or CHISs, and beyond. The quality assurance equation is a good example. Early work on standards, identification of records, and security provides building blocks for CPRs and data repositories, which in turn are building blocks for developing guidelines for community use.

Healthcare executives are encouraged to follow the recommendations concerning the national environment for CHINs by working with national groups themselves, and encouraging their professional and information technology staffs to do so as well, to implement programs with real healthcare value. The opportunity to participate in, for example, nationally based high-risk and specialty networks adds incentives for enterprise participation and CHIN maturation. Professional staff also should welcome the opportunity to participate in a well-funded collegial research program that relies on sharing hot-off-the-press patient information.

State and national lawmaking bodies are introducing healthcare legislation in record amounts. The legislation covers the gamut from requirements for standards, confidentiality, accountability for quality of care, demonstration projects, proof or evaluation of technology, and improving access to telecommunications, to curbing managed care excesses and dictating medical care processes. Healthcare executives are urged to help initiate and support legislation that will bring us closer to the ideal healthcare system we need and to speak out against that which does not.

Much is wrong with healthcare today, and many of the current pressures on the system are making it worse. The system is professionally and administratively rudderless, at the mercy of market forces at the highest levels. Billions of dollars have been taken from the system as profit—dollars that might have been available for strengthening the system's infrastructure. The tobacco and oil industries have each recently given us examples of courageous corporate executives who have chosen publicly to break ranks with their industries when they have acted contrary to the best interests of the societies they serve. Healthcare executives are urged to do the same.

References

Benton International. 1994. *Planning Guide for Community Health Management Information Systems.* New York: The John A. Hartford Foundation.

Hammond, W. E. 1997. "Call for a Standard Clinical Vocabulary." *Journal of the American Medical Informatics Association* 4 (3): 254–55.

Weed, L. L. 1993. "Medical Records That Guide and Teach." *M.D. Computing* 10 (2): 110–14. (Originally published in 1968.)

Glossary

Building Block Analysis. A technique for identifying healthcare goals and start-up CHIN capabilities that are compatible and realistic. A bottom analysis determines whether planned CHIN capabilities are indeed building blocks toward healthcare goals. A top-down analysis specifies capabilities that are building blocks for agreed-upon goals.

Building blocks. CHIN components and capabilities that clearly and directly contribute to, and are essential to, the goals of the CHIN.

Central data repository (CDR). A database in which patient information is stored for such future purposes as quality assurance programs, accreditation, and clinical research. All or a portion of a patient's record may exist in multiple CDRs serving different purposes or different locations.

Centralized network. A telecommunications network in which a single, multipurpose mainframe computer stores all information, provides all services, and carries out all CHIN functions. CHIN components would communicate with each other through the mainframe computer instead of directly. See client server network.

Client server network. A distributed telecommunications network that allows multiple clients (users) to communicate with multiple servers (special purpose computers) at will. See centralized network.

Community health information network (CHIN). A specialized health information network designed to meet healthcare-related information needs for a community. A key feature is participation by multiple community enterprises, for mutually defined healthcare purposes.

Community health information system (CHIS). A mature CHIN that is integrated into the healthcare system.

Community information service center (CISC). A CHIN component that manages a specific complex information flow task or resource such as a CDR or a CMPI.

Community master patient index (CMPI). A database that contains information about the location and identification of patient records for all residents of a community.

Compensatory dissonance. New problems that arise as a consequence of actions taken to solve initial problems.

Computer-based patient record (CPR). An electronically available record of a person's complete medical history and case management across multiple locations, providers, and dates. The term is also currently used to refer to any portion of the patient record that is electronically available, especially claims processing information.

Database. An electronically available set of records.

Enterprise. Any organization involved in providing for healthcare, including such entities as doctors' offices, clinics, hospitals, outpatient facilities, home care agencies, skilled nursing facilities, payors, integrated delivery systems, educational institutions, and research institutions, in any combination.

Enterprise network. A health information network that links multiple locations and functions for and within a single enterprise.

Enterprise standards of care. Clinical guidance that is based heavily on studies of the clinical experience of patients treated at a single enterprise.

Firewall. Software that resides on a server (computer) connected to the Internet, for the purpose of protecting its CHIN operations and information from intrusions by other Internet users. This server on which the firewall resides would typically be the only point of contact between the CHIN and the Internet.

Health information network (HIN). An integrated, interactive information technology-based network designed to meet information needs for the healthcare system. It includes not only hardware, software, storage, and retrieval and electronic communications capabilities, but also the processes, rules, and safeguards necessary for effective support of the healthcare system.

Information block. A situation where information exists, such as in patient records or in the medical knowledge base, but is not available for practical use.

Information technology. Hardware, software, and telecommunications capabilities combined to create information systems.

Infrastructure. The supporting framework of a system that enables it to fulfill its mission. The infrastructure of healthcare would include not only physical facilities for delivering care, but also the capability to do resource planning, educate professionals, transmit information, and conduct the research necessary for the provision of healthcare.

Infostructure. The information infrastructure required to deliver the information flows needed by the healthcare system.

Internet. A collection of telecommunications networks throughout the world that are linked together to offer limited, easy-to-use telecommunications capabilities to everyone, including businesses, governments, educational institutions, and individuals.

Intranet. A private telecommunications network of any size and scope, with restricted access, that uses the same user-friendly technology as the Internet.

Quality assurance. Its two components are quality assessment, which measures the current status of the quality of healthcare at an institution or in the system, and quality acquisition, which comprises the actions that can be taken to impart or assure quality, including curriculum reform, continuing medical education, clinical guidelines, and access to knowledge sources.

Master patient index (MPI). A database, usually belonging to an enterprise, containing information about the location and identification of all of a patient's medical records.

Medical knowledge base (MKB). The totality of medical knowledge, which exists in many forms and locations.

Population standards of care. Clinical guidance that is based on studies of the clinical experiences of large and representative numbers of patients.

Stakeholder. Any community enterprise or group participating in or affected by a CHIN. Examples are providers, payors, patients, local businesses, schools, and government agencies.

Systems perspective. The facility of examining the interactions of all aspects of a system, and the system as a whole, in an attempt to understand the system.

Telemedicine. Remote delivery of healthcare through telecommunications facilities, including doctor-patient audio- and video-communication, instrumentation, and imaging.

Value-added service provider. A contracted organization that provides integrative capabilities, analyses, management, and other services for complex CHIN applications that are beyond the scope of a CHIN to accomplish otherwise.

Value Assessment. A technique for determining and displaying the relevance of planned CHIN capabilities to healthcare goals.

Index

About the Author

KAREN A. DUNCAN is a planning consultant and writer with 30 years of experience in healthcare information systems. She holds a doctorate in Biostatistics from the University of Oklahoma Medical Center and she is the author or editor of over 60 publications, including *Health Information and Health Reform: Understanding the Need for a National Health Information System.*